Deadly Negligence

(Prayer, Trust, Believe, Miracles)

How PaviElle was brought back from DEATH
After hospital SCREW UP

Diana Wright

Deadly Negligence
(Prayer, Trust, Believe, Miracles)

How PaviElle was brought back from DEATH
After hospital SCREW UP

A True Story

By

Diana Wright

Copyright© Diana Wright–February 10, 2012. All rights reserved. No part of this book may be reproduced or retransmitted in any form or by any means without the expressed written permission of the publisher.

Cover design: Christie Designs
Text pages design: Huntley Burgher
Photography for front and back covers: Jay Gayle
Edited by: Dr. Garth Rose

IISBN-13: 978-1495440397
ISBN-10: 1495440397

Printed in the United States of America

Except in the United States of America, this book is sold subject to the condition that it shall not, by way of trade or otherwise, be lent, re-sold, hired out, or otherwise circulated without the publisher's prior consent in any form of binding or cover other than that in which it is published and without a similar condition including this condition being imposed on the subsequent purchaser.

Dedication

To my sweet daughter PaviElle, and all the families, or individuals, who have endured the raging storm that blew through their lives as the result of medical malpractice either by a physician, nurse or hospital, or all of them combined. With courage, perseverance, God's GRACE and FAVOR you are being restored, and totally healed creatively with continued prayer, faith and believing, with unwavering trust in the LORD.

"In his favor is life: weeping may endure for a night but joy cometh in the morning." - Psalm 30:5

May this joy perpetuate in your life, despite the challenges.

Introduction

Why are hospitals, doctors and nurses allowed to commit critical medical malpractices that often times maim, or even kill innocent children, putting their loved ones through unnecessary pain suffering, and seem to get away with it?

With their mighty and powerful legal bully arm, when one is bold enough to take legal action related to their inept practices, with no one to answer to, they make ridiculous offers at legal mediation that are downright insulting as they tend to forget your child or loved one, will NEVER be the SAME AGAIN.

When your life is going great, have you ever sat down and thought, that in an instant, for example with a stick of an IV needle by the hand of an uncaring nurse and an unattached doctor, your life as you know it could be GONE?

Never in my wildest dreams or imagination would I have envisioned that this could happen in my life and least of all to my PERFECT ONLY CHILD, PaviElle Devareaux.

Nine months later in the midst of PaviElle's miraculous recovery, my

In writing this book, which has been difficult and emotionally draining, as the memories are rehashed, reappearing with every stroke of my pen on these pages, I pray deeply, that my story will help families prepare their minds, as they face the unexpected and seemingly impossible events that could occur in their lives.

My hope is that this book will help someone, somewhere in the world, to BELIEVE in MIRACLES. Know that though you walk through the "valley of the shadow of death" you will fear no evil for GOD is always with you. He will bring you through your deepest darkest moments and bring complete healing and restoration to your situation and life. This you will receive through your FAITH, and by BELIEVING when you PRAY.

Acknowledgements

In writing this book I have cried many buckets of tears because of rehashing the memories of this extremely desolate dark hole in my daughter's and my life.

Sharing the story is our testimony of how good God is and how he continues to perform miracles. It is strange how some people say they don't believe in miracles until they need one. Remember, we are never interested in our neighbor's blazing fire until the fire is in our house.

As I took this devastating journey that I had to claim as my tsunami with seemingly endless waves, I must thank God for the angel he sent into my life in the form of Prophetess Dr. Charmaine Peart. She always seemed to know from a distance exactly when she needed to call me, just before I would begin to fall into that deep dark place of depression and tears. She became my pastor and counselor.

Dr. Brina Rubin was there from the beginning and was so faithful in using her Sabbath to visit the hospital more than an hour away. She always brought something, whether it was food for me, a book to read to PaviElle, or someone like her friend Claudina who so reminded to PaviElle. This he did to stimulate her reading and comprehension skills, with every session ending with a prayer.

Roberta, my neighbor, and Ms. Parrado, PaviElle's guidance counselor, who shared their personal stories of their brain injuries with me. They did it so I could have hope and hang on, knowing that PaviElle would recover but it would take time.

To all the therapists in Florida and Atlanta, nurses and doctors, who participated in what they knew in their hearts, was a grave error of malpractice on the part of colleagues, I say thank you all.

I must single out physical therapist Janet Michaels who gave us so much hope, encouragement and dedication. She located the institution in Atlanta that would give PaviElle the biggest boost of intense therapy that she needed to propel her recovery.

Maureen, the nurse at Jackson Memorial Hospital, who gave me whatever I needed for PaviElle to heal as I continued taking care of my sweet girl. She took the time to read through my daughter's file after listening to my account of the events at the hospital and gave me priceless advice that I acted upon.

Loretta, the nurse in Atlanta, who I could call any time and all our needs would be taken care of.

My aunt Lucille, who took her vacation to come and sleep at the hospital one night so I could go home and have one good night of

Prologue

PaviElle, my daughter, was the result of a planned pregnancy and her birth was filled with joy and expectation. Although she did not turn to the right position for delivery, my trusted friend and OBGYN Dr. Jean Chin brought her into the world by Cesarean Section.

Life for baby PaviElle was good and her pediatrician constantly said she only came to her for her regular shots as she was never sick.

On the day she was born our bond was sealed when my husband brought her close to my face for a kiss. She held my thumb and squeezed it so tight I asked the doctor where she got such strength. At the time I did not know she would need that solid strength to bring her back from the edge of death.

When I named her everyone was surprised at the unusual name, saying that spelling it would be challenging. However, I considered the name, one that would give special presence whenever PaviElle Devareaux enters a room, or said her name.

All parents say their child is beautiful, but believe me; PaviElle was very beautiful before her tragic illness, and an absolutely gorgeous, in Miami, Florida. She was smart and a very good student, making the Principal's list in 5th grade at Kipp Academy, a school that really challenged her mind. Students would be calling every night asking for her help with homework and she never said no.

As she moved to middle school her ability continued to excel in Math. She also excelled in Spanish, with almost a perfect Spanish accent. Her reward was winning awards in drama competitions, and being the narrator of the Spanish play at the end of the school year.

I enrolled her in golf and tennis where she impressed the coaches of both games. The golf instructor told us to prepare for a golf scholarship and the tennis instructor encouraged me to get her a private coach, as she had real potential. She felt great and wanted to pursue both sports with gusto. Unfortunately, PaviElle's life journey was derailed in devastation and despair in her thirteenth year, when taking a full dose of Amoxicillin, an antibiotic which gave an allergic reaction of extreme proportions that triggered an autoimmune disease called Juvenile Rheumatoid Arthritis (JRA).

Foreword

When PaviElle attended middle school I was not one of her teachers, yet, it was very rapidly that I met the family through its deep commitment to the school and the academic experiences of PaviElle . I served as the Parent Liaison working to increase parental involvement and PaviElle's mother was one of our pillars. We formed a bond borne of a deep appreciation I had for the family, given the time and effort they contributed to our school life.

It was like a lightning strike when after school was out for the summer I received a call at my home as I prepared dinner. Mrs. McLaughlin had my cell number, and called to say she was at a Palm Beach hospital where her daughter was fighting for her life and that no one from the school had called or visited. I ran out of the house, leaving the stove top burner on.

At the hospital room I was shaken to find PaviElle seemingly unresponsive and hooked up to assorted medical equipment. PaviElle was a ravishing slender young lady, poised, tall, bright, and extremely beautiful. Friends and teachers alike were always drawn to her. Her warmth, loving nature, and overall demeanor were very apparent and she was a people magnet, truly. Scholastically she was a journey into the darkness? What comes to mind is Henry Ford's words: Obstacles are those frightful things you see when you take your eyes off your goal. Mrs. McLaughlin never took her eyes off the goal but dealt with the obstacles like a dragon slayer. Mrs. McLaughlin was a TV personality and a most accomplished professional in her native island, and was on the cusp of starting a new career in the States when catastrophe struck. Now all revolved around saving PaviElle from the clutches of utter destruction. It was a monumental fight of a lifetime, with endless battles constantly popping up from obtaining medical care, to services, and to a diet that if left to the system's wisdom would have destroyed Pavi who had a history of distinct food allergens. From a national media star to a warrior for the salvation of her child, Mrs. McLaughlin's transformation was nothing less than stunning.

The medical prognosis was devastating, and decisively hopeless. Mrs. McLaughlin believed otherwise. What man cannot, God can, she said. The array of Herculean tasks was daunting, transferring Pavi from the hospital setting to the house, first reviving the physical functions, then addressing the slow and painful return to normal emotional and cognitive normalcy, and then the trip to another state for further rehabilitation. Mrs. McLaughlin tirelessly engaged the best professionals one could find for the various needs of PaviElle, from speech, occupational and physical therapists, to nutritionists and neurologists, and finally to academicians. The circle of help which Mrs. McLaughlin created was beyond belief. Nothing could stop her in obtaining that which was declared unobtainable. As the saying goes, she did the impossible first and then the difficult.

jobs call for big measures. Yet, I saw a mother use a dropper, if you will, to turn a desert into a garden. PaviElle's story is astounding, as is her family.

Brina I. Rubin, Ed.D.

Chapter 1

*I*f you love someone set them free. If they come back they are meant to be yours; if they don't they were never yours. This is what I did years ago when I gave up my one true love that came back to me in a strange coincidence.

Early in my broadcast and journalism career I soared in my success being a nightly TV news anchor, then the youngest and only female news director, and the greatest of them all. Later I became the creator, producer and anchor of my own TV show, the "Diana Wright Show." This would become the most watched television show in my native country, Jamaica, and also popular in London and Florida.

In my quest to achieve all this, I found my lost love again after taking a crushed message slip from the garbage bin in my office. On that slip of paper was written the name Lloyd. To my surprise I soon learned he, like myself, was back in Jamaica, saw my picture on the front page of the Sunday magazine of a leading newspaper and decided to find me. As his story goes, he stopped by my office and was told I was out of the country so he left a message. When I returned my assistant had crushed the paper and put it in the garbage. It must have been a miracle that I decided to remove the paper and saw

Life had been great until TRAGEDY struck with our sweet girl.

On the day she was born our bond was sealed when my husband brought her close to my face for a kiss. She held my thumb and squeezed it so tight I asked the doctor where she got such strength. At the time I did not know she would need that solid strength to bring her back from the edge of death.

When I named her everyone was surprised at the unusual name, saying that spelling it would be challenging. However, I considered the name, one that would give special presence whenever PaviElle Devareaux enters a room, or said her name.

All parents say their child is beautiful, but believe me; PaviElle was very beautiful before her tragic illness, and an absolutely gorgeous, kind, sensitive, well behaved and respectful child. I remember her guidance counselor Ms. Parrado in Middle school saying, PaviElle was 13 years old and behaved just like a 13 year old.

Everywhere we went she was admired by strangers, especially for her very long hair, all of which she lost at Jackson Memorial Hospital in Miami, Florida. She was smart and a very good student, making the Principal's list in 5th grade at Kipp Academy, a school that really challenged her mind. Students would be calling every night asking for her help with homework and she never said no.
As she moved to middle school her ability continued to excel in Math. She also excelled in Spanish, with almost a perfect Spanish accent. Her reward was winning awards in drama competitions, and

pursue both sports with gusto. Unfortunately, PaviElle's life journey was derailed in devastation and despair.

The nightmare of PaviElle's and my life began on May 25, 2007 when I took her for a MRI to examine the swollen glands on the right side of her neck, just below her ear. This test was ordered by her rheumatologist who finally listened to my persistent cries that she was allergic to the medication Kineret.

After the test was done we left the Palm Beach hospital both feeling happy and even stopped at Dunkin Doughnuts for a treat. PaviElle was full of joy as we journeyed back home on that beautiful sunny day in Palm Beach County, Florida, with fluffy white clouds in the sky. Unfortunately, our feeling of euphoria and relief came to an abrupt end after a call from the rheumatologist.

He first apologized for giving me bad news on the phone, but said he received the MRI results and it seemed PaviElle had lymphoma, a form of cancer. I rejected this news, and again told him I thought it was the Kineret that was causing the swelling of the lymph-nodes because I had read this was a possible symptom in the literature that came with the medication. He basically ignored me and said he had taken the liberty to make an appointment with Dr. Anexas an oncologist/hematologist at the hospital. He also said the good news was that the treatment for Lymphoma would cure the Juvenile Rheumatic Arthritis (JRA). At that crushing moment I thought why did he not use that treatment to cure the JRA, that seem to attack so many of his patients, instead of the ridiculous cocktail of drugs given

When I got off the telephone I noticed PaviElle's breathing seemed labored, her pulse fast and blood pressure low. I quickly called the doctor back and he instructed me to take her to, what would become to me, the "Hospital of Death," which, unfortunately, I am not allowed to name because of a gag order from the eventual malpractice lawsuit we filed. It can only be referred to as a hospital in Palm Beach County.

When we arrived at the hospital, the usual paper work was done and we were placed in a room from 3:30 p.m. to 10:30 p.m. I kept saying to myself, "If someone comes here and is really dying, they certainly would, after waiting so long."

They finally did an X-Ray of PaviElle's chest and a cat scan. I was very shocked when the radiologist asked me who was taking care of my daughter as he looked at the results. He simply said in a low voice, "They should be shot". At that moment I knew all my maternal instincts about PaviElle's illness were right. She was admitted, and we settled in for the night on the oncology floor of the hospital.

On June 7, 2007 I watched my only child dying as she sat on the bedside commode, then on her hospital bed, but God gave her back to us one MIRACLE at a time.

Approximately three years later, March 10, 2010 at 2:30 p.m., as I waited for PaviElle to come out of school, with tears running down my face I wrote this.

Through this storm I know

Deadly Negligence

> *I Trust you Lord*
> *I need and depend on you everyday*
> *With open heart and hands*
> *To receive your every Blessing*
> *For Total and Complete Recovery for PaviElle*

I constantly keep in my mind the words of my mother as she tries to encourage me, *"Rejoice not over me mine enemies, for though I fall I'll rise again."*

I kept feeling, as I watched my daughter travel close to death, and the dire struggles she encountered in her very young life, as if my life had been hit and torpedoed by the combination of a tsunami, hurricane, tornado and an earthquake. I kept asking silently, and aloud, "Why?" I still am not quite sure I have the answer but I know that with God, through his son Jesus, I weathered and triumphed over it, and will continue to do so. Romans 8:28 says and this I know to be true, *"All things work together for good to them that love God; to them who are called according to his purpose."* I have to remind myself on the days that are hard beyond explanation that; *"With God all things are possible,"* Matthew 19:26

The day I knew for sure that in Christ alone my hope would be found is when Claudina, a woman who truly reminded me of Mother Teresa prayed with me at PaviElle's bedside as she laid swollen like an inflated balloon with helium in the Pediatric Intensive Care Unit (PICU) isolation room at Jackson Memorial Hospital, Claudina said to me, "Don't worry; you will see miraculous changes in 4 days." As the power of His love and my love for my only child PaviElle. The popular song with the words, "In the arms of the angels may you find some comfort here," Also this became a constant motivator in my broken heart.

When tragedy hits your life you learn very quickly that you don't need much to survive. As I slept on the hard bench at the hospital for almost six months watching my only child lay still in a coma I realized that having only three panties that I washed nightly, hoping they would dry in the morning, material things meant absolutely nothing. Seeing the person you love and cherish most in life lay seemingly DEAD was all that consumed my mind, soul and body.

June 7, 2007 at 4:00 a.m. will be etched in my memory for the rest of my life. It was the day a nurse refused to listen to my adamant refusal to give PaviElle the medication, Versed. I knew PaviElle should not have the medication, but the nurse ignored my pleas and gave it to her anyway, and helplessly, I watched as my single most cherished responsibility sat on a bedside commode dying as I screamed for help and no one came. That morning I did my best to clean her up but her body became heavier and heavier. Finally getting her back into bed, her body became cold and washed with sweat at the same time. I screamed, "She's dying. PaviElle is dying. I told you not to give her the Versed." I became more panicked, intense and louder, but still no nurse responded to my cries.

Almost a year into PaviElle's recovery and intense rehabilitation my life would experience another tsunami. I got a call on my cell convinced and kept thinking about the Bible, and the account in the book of Genesis when Joseph kept having recurring dreams which were eventually revealed as the truth.

After thanking her for the information I asked God how much more would he give me? I have quickly learned that the sub-title of my book, PRAYER, TRUST, BELIEVE equals MIRACLES is on point.

Each and every day since that disastrous incident on June 7, 2007 I have experienced a journey that I would not wish on my worst enemy, but am so thankful for the miracles I have been given every single day as PaviElle's normal life is restored. As I took this journey, make no mistake, I questioned God numerous times and was even angry at Him sometimes. I kept asking how He could have made this consuming tragedy happen to someone as special as my daughter. I would ask, "God, you are supernatural and gave me such a blessing with PaviElle, So why God, why does it seem like she is slipping away?"

But, then I would also answer my own question, telling myself, "Diana, you have enjoyed 13 beautiful years with her."

Chapter 2

ooking back to where it all began with PaviElle's diagnosis of Juvenile Rheumatoid Arthritis (JRA) by a rheumatologist who had the most horrible bedside manner, we were thrown into a toxic world of poisonous medication cocktails.

If only my friend of over 30 years, had shared her daughter's diagnosis with the same autoimmune disease, where she was told to go home and take aspirins, PaviElle's tragic experience might have been prevented.

After a brief hospital stay for a battery of tests, some unnecessary in my opinion, the devastating journey began. A second rheumatologist entered our lives with a more extensive, rigorous cocktail of medication but a better demeanor.

His prescription of the drug cocktail seemed so extreme I resisted, only to be reprimanded and threatened by him to be reported to the Department of Children and Families, if I did not allow PaviElle to be given the medication. Although the medication began to show an extreme allergic reaction on her glands, he still insisted that she would be a good day but my heart was actually uneasy because she was not feeling well. She was extremely quiet and not eating much. My tense anticipation of the MRI results for her swollen glands may not have been obvious, but my nervous energy seemed to fill the atmosphere.

As she got dressed for school I noticed her movements were very slow and labored. Her effervescent personality seemed to have vanished, so I hugged her tight trying to give her the reassurance she would soon feel much better, and, honestly, even in my fast beating heart, I thought she would snap out of it and be well again.

As we prepared to leave for her school the sound of a car in my driveway un-nerved me, but I was mistaken it was a car in my Neighbor's driveway. Immediately after I left to take PaviElle to her school, feeling extremely nervous.

Our journey to school, a short distance away, seemed to take forever. I knew she should have stayed home, but PaviElle with her love for school insisted on going. Turning in her completed Math project was extremely important to her so I accommodated her decision to attend classes.

As we got to school, I could see her fading into a weak, slow moving person but she was persistent. God made us run into Mr. Bishop, her Math teacher, and as we handed him the project he noticed PaviElle was not feeling well. He was very caring and told her not to worry, but, on the other hand, her science teacher was totally insensitive, heard a car in the driveway, and this time I was right as it was a friend who worked in the medical field.

When she came into the house, she noticed how sick PaviElle looked and decided to take her pulse and blood pressure. As she was doing this, the telephone rang. It was the rheumatologist calling with the results of the MRI that was done a few days earlier. He insisted that PaviElle might have lymphoma and I kept saying no, she was allergic to the cocktail of medication that he prescribed.

Mother's intuition triumphed as we went to the hospital and all tests including neck biopsy and a bone marrow test showed reaction to the medications. As all the expert doctors came with their varied misdiagnosis, and completely ignored what I was telling them, my daughter's condition seemed more puzzling to me.

As the panic escalated we were quickly moved to pediatric ICU where everything just appeared to be descending into a very deep dark hole of devastation. It all came to a disastrous place after the head-honcho Doctor told me off earlier in the day so I was alert. At approximately 4:00 a.m. after a nurse ignored my pleas and persisted in giving PaviElle Chlora Hydrate and Versed although I had insisted that she should not be given any more medication for the night. While I had my daughter on the bedside commode trying to comfort her, the same evil nurse came into the room, hiding the needle with the Versed. I adamantly refused to let her give the medication, but she still stuck it into the IV line. It had an instantaneous effect. In a moment I watched my only child dying before my eyes. I asked the

the potty, as she became extremely heavy, her eyes rolling over and she was looking like a dead person.

As my anxiety rose, I struggled to put her back in bed then went to the door of her room screaming on the top of my lungs at 'Nurse Death' asking, "What did you give my child? She looks like she's DEAD. I told you not to give her anything else. I told you to write a note to Dr. Jerk that I refused the medication and still you gave it to my child anyway."

At this point she told me she had written a note to the doctor. Then virtually ignoring me, the nurse simply continued to sit at her desk writing notes preparatory to the ending of her shift. By the time I went back into the room PaviElle was cold and sweating profusely at the same time. Again I started screaming, "She's cold and sweaty, you killed my kid."

Even at my obvious panic at the sight of PaviElle's plight, 'Nurse Death' and the respiratory therapist kept telling me she needed to get the medicine because she needed to sleep and rest her lungs. While they were trying to explain this nonsense to me, I just kept saying, "Can't you see my child is dying?" I continued to protest, repeatedly telling the respiratory therapist, "I told the nurse not to give PaviElle the Versed. Why didn't she listen to me?" The respiratory therapist decided to check PaviElle's blood after a very long time. As I watched her draw the blood, I could see she was trying to hide the panic in her face. She then said to me, "I need to get a new kit because I don't like what I am seeing." As she left the room, I could feel my heart kid." At this point the RT then tried to wake up PaviElle by slapping her face, but she could not wake up. She pressed the button above the bed and PaviElle then CODED. This is something that you never want to hear, especially as a parent. She had gone into CARDIAC

More Panic ensued and everyone came running from everywhere in the hospital trying to resuscitate PaviElle. They threw me out of the room, but I kept screaming what had become my chant, "I told her not to give PaviElle the Versed, she killed my kid." Some of the nurses tried to console me, but I just kept repeating my chant. I called my husband and sister-in-law, telling them to come, because they killed PaviElle, but if they had listened to me this would not have happened.

As the medical team completed their effort to resuscitate her, her body was swollen and she no longer looked like my beautiful, sweet girl. The hospital management decided to transfer her to Jackson Memorial Hospital in Miami. However, the hospital personnel, headed by Dr. Jerk, had great difficulty getting PaviElle to be airlifted to this other hospital because there was no bed available in that hospital's pediatric Intensive care unit (PICU).

Finally, after several long hours, the helicopter arrived and PaviElle was bundled and strapped into it and taken to Jackson Memorial Hospital. My husband and I had to drive an hour and a half to Miami because there was no room in the helicopter for both, or either, of us. Our journey was tense and filled with anxiety and anticipation as clean bill of health. He insisted she continue taking the Kineret that I ferociously refused and then later scolded and threatened me that he would no longer be her doctor if I did not do the bone marrow test ordered by Dr. Anexas. My emotions ran wild as my heart raced like something ready to erupt like a volcano. I distinctly remembered the morning when Dr. Anexas came to see us and explained the process of the various tests to rule out lymphoma. I recalled that as I listened my intuition kept saying, PaviElle does NOT have lymphoma. All that was happening was that she was showing the side effects of Kineret and the extensive cocktail of medication that were explained in the pamphlet that came with the medicines. "Why are these doctors not listening to me?" I asked myself. "Are they just determined to bill Medicaid for unnecessary tests?"

Chapter 3

During the long drive to Miami, I recounted all that had taken place that day. After PaviElle was admitted the doctors started with a biopsy of the swollen glands behind PaviElle's right ear, then a bone marrow test and finally an open biopsy of one of the lymph-nodes. While we nervously waited, the surgeon, Dr. Stone, who would perform the surgery for the open biopsy came to the room and discussed the situation.

He explained that since PaviElle was having respiratory problems he was not comfortable giving her anesthesia to do the open biopsy, so he would prefer to wait. I agreed completely, because the respiratory problem was one of the main reasons that I took PaviElle to the

Finally, I felt a doctor was listening to me about my child's illness, its progression and my concern about the drugs being prescribed for her. After that conversation, Dr. Anexas decided to give PaviElle the first Biopsy. The procedure was done, and with cheers, clapping hands and hugs from the nurses as we returned to the floor, I was told, "Mom, you were right; the results are negative for lymphoma full steam ahead and do the bone marrow test. I told him, I would have to discuss the situation with my husband and my sister-in-law, Sharon, who is a registered nurse.

After we held this discussion we decided to refuse the test because we did not believe PaviElle had lymphoma. Dr. Anexas became very annoyed and irate with me, saying we would have to be discharged from the hospital and go somewhere else because we were refusing the test. He stormed out of the room declaring he would call Dr. Namdoog, the rheumatologist.

At that juncture, I decided to go home, take a shower and change my clothes. On my way Dr. Namdoog called, and he was furious. He said I was "pissing off" the doctors, at the Hospital of Death. He kept insisting the bone marrow test must be done to rule out lymphoma and I kept asking him about the information that came with the medication Kineret that clearly clarified the symptoms PaviElle was having. He refused to listen to me, so I told him to call my husband and after he did, and under complete duress we decided to do the test.

It seemed God was sending a message to delay the bone marrow test because one of the nurses, Denisia, gave PaviElle Morphine without my consent. When I asked why she had done that, she gave some stupid explanation that her blood pressure was low and the drug would relax her heart. I had done some research to confirm what I was thinking about the medications and my thoughts were logical, as I evaluated what this nurse was telling me. How could PaviElle

With all of this going on, I was shocked to see Dr. Anexas again scheduling the bone marrow test. I began to wonder if he got more pay to do this test. He consulted with the anesthesiologist and she was great. She took a very long time to talk with me because she knew I did not want the test to be done, and had great concerns about it being done while PaviElle was having respiratory problems. She assured me that the Versed she was giving her to sedate her for the procedure would be closely watched by her, and to make me more at ease she would move PaviElle from the regular procedure room to the regular operating room. Somehow, I felt better, as she showed me the tube with the amount of Versed that would be injected.

The test was done and again the result was NEGATIVE. I now wondered, what was the next diagnosis they would pull out of their hats, instead of addressing the one that I was only concerned about the respiratory problem. This was the main reason I took her to the emergency room in the first place.

Soon after the bone marrow test, PaviElle was up and cheerful, asking for food. This brought joy and warmth to my heart, so I called my mom and let her speak to PaviElle who told her grandmother, "I'm fine Grandma." I asked the nurse if it was okay for her to eat the meal that was served. She checked with 'Dr. Aloof' who said it was safe for her to eat before taking her medication. She ate a banana and half of a chicken wing, and seemed fine. She then took the cocktail of medication, went to sleep and woke up asking for the chicken. I smiled and told her it had been taken away. She asked to use the potty, and after laying down a while began to have problems me that the doctor had left something for her to sleep so if I wanted her to get it let her know. I again explained to 'Nurse Death,' that PaviElle had anesthesia for the bone marrow test during the day and a lot of other medication so I did not think her body could handle any more drugs. I told her I would stay up with her until she falls asleep. I guess that was not a good reasoning for her, because the nurse simply wanted her to go to sleep and stop moaning. She kept coming back several times, trying to convince me that I needed to sleep and PaviElle needed to take the drugs to sleep. Finally, she came back with a syringe and explained that it was a mild sedative called Chlora Hydrate, given to babies. It would not hurt her and be easy to take, with a squeeze into her mouth. I told her I was not comfortable with any medication to be given to my daughter to help her sleep, but she could go ahead and give the Chlora Hydrate, but nothing else. Needless to say this did not work, just as I thought it wouldn't.

But, 'Nurse Death' was about to pounce into action, catching me off guard while PaviElle was on the bedside commode. She came in with her hand behind her back with yet another syringe. This time it would be the DEADLY ONE. She injected it into the IV and I got very irate and screamed at her, "Did I tell you not to give her anything else, how can you give Chlora Hydrate at 2:00 a.m. and give her Versed two hours later?" 'Nurse Death' left the room without an answer and in another few moments I could not lift PaviElle off the potty. She became very heavy, her eyes rolling over and she looked like a dead person. I struggled to put PaviElle in bed and went to the door screaming at 'Nurse Death,' asking, "Why did you give her same drug the anesthesiologist gave for the bone marrow procedure and took so many precautions. Instantly I knew this was wrong, especially after I told 'Nurse Death' so many times not to give anymore medication.

By the time I got back to her bedside, PaviElle was cold and sweating at the same time. I started screaming, "She is cold and sweating you killed my kid." I kept replaying this in my mind every time I had a free moment to think.

After all the confusion following the cardiac arrest, Dr. Aloof finally arrived and had the nerve to say she was going to put PaviElle on the ventilator after the bone marrow procedure but heard she had eaten chicken. I could not believe my ears because before I gave her the chicken, the nurse told me she had to check with the doctor, and she had come back and said the doctor said she could eat, especially since she would be given her medication.

Before I left for Miami, the nurse who had taken PaviElle to the OR had the nerve to say to me, "Don't be doctor, just be mom." I was too distraught to really tell her what was in my heart after my only child almost died in their hospital.

Chapter 4

Arriving at Jackson Memorial gave me hope, mixed with trepidation, as we were received By Dr. Bukas and Nurse Domingo. They seemed a compassionate team, in comparison to the uncaring personnel and chaotic scenario we left behind. Almost immediately, Dr. Bukas's first concern was there could be brain injury after the cardiac arrest at the Palm Beach hospital. He ordered a brain scan stat, which at the time seemed clear. This was good news for the medical team, but in my heart and with my mother's intuition I knew, looking at PaviElle, that the news was wrong. I then decided to rely on my Faith, Belief and Trust in God, drilled by My grandmother, Henereta Gordon, from I was a little girl.

After a very long and exhausting wait for a diagnosis, the rheumatologist called the intensivist at Jackson Memorial with another one. Only this time, it was a name so rare, no one was able to clearly explain the details. This new scary diagnosis was MICROPHAGE ACTIVATION SYNDROME, but to confirm this new alien, an open biopsy of the lymph node under PaviElle's left arm had to be done to again rule out lymphoma 100 percent. "Oh, my God," I thought, how many times, are the doctors going to test to rule out lymphoma. "Did the

PaviElle's feet and hands had become black, plus there was a major black wound on her right thigh. With a racing heart, I asked Dr. McLaughlin what that meant? She said with a visible sad face, that the black coloring and wound was caused because of the cardiac arrest and lack of circulation that took place at the Palm Beach hospital. The next day her lips were extremely swollen and Dr. McLaughlin explained that PaviElle was allergic to a medication she had been given to her earlier, but which was stopped immediately. Finally, the rare and deadly diagnosis was confirmed. PaviElle had Microphage Activation Syndrome, MAS. We were given a pile of paper, with information taken from the internet. I immediately went outside to the waiting room and read the entire material, then pursued my own research and was stunted by the rarity of this autoimmune disease.

The doctor carefully explained the treatment process that included steroids and the big gun - CHEMOTHERAPY VC16. The most devastating news came next, when Dr. Navez did another test called a lumbar puncture on PaviElle to check if her brain was damaged by the cardiac arrest, or the MAS diagnosis. The results of the lumbar puncture did not rule out brain injury one hundred percent, therefore another test, an MRI, needed to be done.

The killer news was delivered on Friday June 22, 2007. The MRI showed the OCIPITAL and TEMPRAL parts of PaviElle's brain were damaged, and it was not by the MAS but caused by the cardiac arrest, and there was nothing that could be done to fix it.
Dr. Selano who gave me this news, had more bad news to give in the afternoon. He said the plastic surgery team had been summoned

Deadly Negligence

about the brain damage caused by the cardiac arrest. Only time would tell, he said.

I gave the MRI results to my sister-in-law Sharon to get a second opinion from the neurologist she worked with. His response provided no hope. He said what happened to PaviElle should never have happened in a PICU in any hospital. He said with the amount of damage to her brain, she would come back with a deficit.

I knew in my heart, that something was severely wrong because PaviElle was not waking up, her entire body was swollen beyond recognition, and everything seemed stacked against her. Despite that low feeling, I knew God would pull her through this valley of the shadow of death. Everyone was hopeless at this point, but me.

Dr. Podda, a mild mannered Italian hematologist/oncologist was my small ray of hope. He was now in charge of PaviElle's chemotherapy V16 treatment. He later added Cyclosporine to the treatment, which he explained was toxic, but could not have been given before, because of the kidney damage caused by the cardiac arrest. This doctor definitely chose the right profession and treated me with great respect.

PaviElle's brain function was still a major concern for the doctors and me, because she was not waking up. The skin on her toes was beginning to break down so an antibiotic ointment was added to help prevent infection. The plastic surgeon eventually came to inspect her various wounds and toes as a result of the cardiac arrest, and the family and friends. Everyone thought I was crazy, but one doctor did say classical music therapy was good for the brain's recovery.

PaviElle's system was now accepting the feed placed in her stomach, being applied through an IV line, placed in her nose, but she was still not waking up or responding to anything. We remained in the isolation room, with everyone having to wear yellow gowns and masks before entering the room. I had to tell Dr. Selena that he should do his job and leave the rest to God because they all seemed so doubtful about PaviElle's recovery. I did believe God would intervene. They kept telling me that only in the movies you see patients with brain injuries wake up from a coma and is totally back to normal, sitting up in their hospital beds.

My first two visitors came and that was the reassurance I needed to contrast with the doom and gloom that surrounded me. These visitors were Dr. Brina Rubin and her friend Claudina, who once had a brain injury, and who had a distinct resemblance, to Mother Theresa. As she prayed and told me about her past brain injury and recovery, I felt the room filled with the Holy Spirit. Before she left the room her words of encouragement to me was, "You'll see a positive change in PaviElle's condition, in four days."

As they left, I wept, but when I turned my head to the left facing the huge window, I saw the brightest, most colorful and defined rainbow. I felt it was so close, I could touch it with my hands, so I dried my tears and went close to PaviElle, kissed her cheek, hugged and whispered in her ear, "Mommy loves you, God loves you and

My relief was crushed when the fever returned after five days but my hope and fighting spirit was unwavering. I decided to put everything into the recovery of my only child and total trust in God.

She was moved from the isolation room for a few days but had to be returned because of fear of infection. At one point I had left the room and she was placed in the open ward, in the Feng Shui death position. I protested vigorously and a wonderful nurse named Maureen moved her to a better position. Her return to isolation released another bout of fear in my heart but I clearly understood the issue of infection being a great concern for the doctors. It is amazing in these hospitals how you are inundated by teams of doctors twice a day.

I overcame the intimidation by doing extensive research of everything the doctors told me, including all medications and their side effects. The doctors were baffled at the questions I would ask; therefore when they changed shifts, the new team would know all about me. Dr. Selena said he went home and thought about me every night and told his wife that he could give me no BS about my daughter's condition because I only wanted the truth. He also told me that throughout his entire career he had seen mothers come to PICU and stayed for a while, some came once in a while, some never came back, but he had never seen another mother like me, who was always there. He told me I had to get some rest so I could be there to take care of PaviElle. I told him not to worry, God was taking care of me, and my mom always said, "You are strongest at your weakest point." He just smiled slightly, shook his head, and tried to convince me that fighting spirit. Along with taking PaviElle off antibiotics, he ordered an ultra sound to look at her kidneys, to see if there is a problem within that was causing her blood pressure to be so high. He also had Nurse Kim remove the catheter and allow PaviElle to pee in a diaper. He changed the dose of Norvast and then gave me his lecture. He said, "There is a possibility that the MAS can be cured and the rehab here at Jackson is very good. For the brain there is nothing I can give to fix it, but with time anything is possible. She will not be 100 percent like she used to be, because of the cardiac arrest and lack of

He disagreed with me that the milk product they were feeding PaviElle, was creating mucus, an allergy she has had since birth. He also scheduled PaviElle to be moved from the PICU to the regular oncology floor. I had my trepidations but that would be his decision.

Unfortunately after all Dr. Gilman's changes, PaviElle developed a fever, after not having one for five days. When Nurse Janice broke the news to me, I kept telling myself to keep the Faith for a Miracle of Healing and Cure. The journey of antibiotics began again, with cultures, blood work, testing mouth secretions and the entire regiment of other tests.

Dr. Gilman also ordered physical and occupational therapy, which gave me a boost as PaviElle was finally moved to a huge chair and sitting up propped with pillows and me hovering over her as if I was preventing her from breaking. At this point she was no longer swollen like an inflated balloon but looked more like someone was offered as the solution, as Dr. George Hernandez and Nurse Janice explained the benefits of the stretched out schedule of the drug.

They assured me that she would be weaned from all drugs, but the withdrawal she was experiencing was normal but uncomfortable. I broke down and cried because her condition looked so scary. I told PaviElle how sorry I was for what she was going through. Janice tried to console me but I could not stop crying. Janice administered the drug and PaviElle calmed down instantly. Janice then got another nurse to change her and made her comfortable for the night.

At this juncture, I was perplexed PaviElle was getting so many drugs and I kept complaining about the effects on that area of her skin where they were inserting the medication with an IV needle. They finally listened to my cries and complaints and Dr. Gilman brought in the PIC line nurse who got my permission to insert the line.

They explained that the PIC line would replace the central line and minimize the risk of infections. It would also serve as a long term catheter, that would be used to draw blood and insert all her medications. They cautioned that there were risks as was the case with every medical procedure, but the central line she had in her upper thigh was more prone to infection. I remember my favorite and trusted nurse, Maureen, telling another nurse that PaviElle should have had a PIC line and the central line taken out. Remembering this, I gave my permission for the procedure to insert the PIC line.

continuously. My success was evident, because all the therapists kept asking me, "Are you doing the therapy twenty four hours a day Mrs. McLaughlin?" I just smiled and kept observing. When PaviElle and I were alone in the room, my system of massage, creaming her skin, rubbing her feet, playing classical music and placing a cold rag on her forehead began to pay off, because she began to sleep peacefully on a regular basis.

As she slept I would take the time to pray and reflect on her progress for the day, then writing it all in my diary. This was necessary because during the day it was so hectic, that there was no time to even take

With all this activity going on, PaviElle remained in a coma, unaware of the chaos around her. I asked the doctors if she could see or hear, as I tried everything possible to get something back. One day I decided to ask her to blink if she knew me and miraculously she BLINKED.

The next day, therapy was great, as PaviElle sat up in the chair in which she was placed with more stability. Nurse Furnede put her arms around me and I cried with joy. Sometimes she opened her eyes and although I knew she most likely was not actually seeing, or comprehending what she saw, I showed PaviElle family albums and she stared at them with intensity. Then I played her favorite movies and television shows repeatedly, and read some of her favorite books aloud. The big joy came, when she opened her mouth for me several times and I tried to make her sip water from a straw. That was not a attentive and gentle they were with PaviElle, were on duty I would sleep at the nearby Ronald McDonald House, the charitable 'home-away-from-home' for family members who have a love one receiving treatment at Jackson Memorial Hospital. But, seeking rest there was really fruitless as all I did was take a shower then kept calling the nurses to check on PaviElle and in the middle of the night I would return to the hospital. Sleep was hard to come for me, as my brain and thoughts were constantly working at rapid speed.

The Ronald McDonald House presented its own dramatic saga. One morning I returned only to find my possessions outside. When I enquired what had happen, I was told the room was needed, since I was not sleeping in it. Devastated, I protested but decided that another fight was not worth it, because I needed all my energy, courage, strength and determination to keep PaviElle restored and alive.

The social worker observed me and decided to help fight my battle because she knew I needed the room especially when my husband Lloyd was able to stay with me. That was very rare, but she insisted and so I accepted her help, although I knew that sleeping on the floor at PaviElle's bedside was the only option that would make me feel comfortable. The doctors and nurses kept pleading with me to get more rest. I certainly needed to get sleep, but I usually told them, "I'm fine." Something strange happened as the chemotherapy, steroids and Cyclosporine regiment continued. Nurse Furnede was removed from PaviElle's care abruptly and replaced with Nurse Bob. PaviElle refused to let Nurse Bob touch her vagina or any part of question why they were giving her a liquid feed with fiber, when all she was taking in was liquids. It was obvious to me that the fiber was the problem. Dr. Watson agreed and the formula was changed.

My anxiety about the chemotherapy and all the other medications escalated, so I insisted on having a meeting with Dr. Podda, the oncologist/hematologist. My favorite nurse, Maureen, arranged the meeting. I explained all my concerns to the doctor indicating that they were similar to my concerns at the hospital in Palm Beach, and he actually listened. We came up with a good solution and he explained everything about the VC16 Chemo, steroids and Cyclosporine, including how the treatment would be scheduled. He also provided me with information about an expert in Sweden, called Dr. Popavitch in Cincinnati, Ohio, and Dr. Kliner, an immunologist at Jackson, and told them about my concerns. I felt very positive about our meeting, and was confident that he had PaviElle's best interest and recovery as a priority.

The next event would be a big one that raised my heart rate and gave me another bout of nervousness like non I experienced before. Dr. Gilman called me into his office to announce that PaviElle's red and white cells and platelets had increased so he was thinking of moving her to the sixth floor of the hospital where Dr. Podda and his team worked, unless something drastic happened for the worst. I asked him about relocating her to the rehab floor, but he said the staff on that floor could not handle the level of medication PaviElle needed, but maybe she could be placed on that floor in another two weeks. I also asked him about the step-down unit, but he said he was not burning questions, that the doctor said she was given that only once a month.

PaviElle was now doing better in therapy and Dr. Gillman decided to eliminate the mask and gown requirement everyone entering the isolation room she occupied had to wear for what seemed like eternity. I thanked the Lord for all His miracles. I told Dr. Hernandez that I wanted to wait before giving PaviElle another dose of VP16 Chemo and to my pleasant surprise Dr. Gillman said one or two nights would not make a difference. That night was the most peaceful night she had since we got to Jackson Memorial Hospital.

As her recovery seemed clearly to be within reach she shocked us by sitting up in the chair from 1:00pm to 8:00pm., thanks to Nurse Dennis. I washed her hair, but could not get all the tangles out, so I twisted it the best I could and she went to bed that night with a blue bonnet on her head. My prayer that night was "God I am waiting for PaviElle's total, one hundred percent, healing through your son Jesus."

PICU Reflection

As I thought about all that had happened to my sweet girl for the past month, my heart grew within my chest, tears filled my eyes and my body that had lost so much weight, seemed very light as I felt the apprehension deep down in my soul. I knew that even though this move from PICU may be a positive one, PaviElle would observed. I then psyched myself and got ready for the next round of battle that I had come so accustomed to.

My reputation as a mother who stayed twenty-four hours a day with her child, and would do and fight for anything that would make her better, obviously preceded us being moved to the sixth floor. I researched everything and requested that she should receive absolutely no medication without my being consulted about side effects and dosage, then giving permission. I recall the plastic surgeon wanting to amputate my child's toes and the rage that engulfed me like an uncontrollable fire towards him and his team. I quickly volunteered to take care of my daughter's feet and hands myself, researching tirelessly to find things good for healing toes that had become so black, only my doubtless belief and trust in God allowed me to see these problems in a positive and healing light.

Chapter 5

On June 30, 2007 PaviElle was moved to the sixth floor, Room 6093A, with the help of my favorite nurse, Maureen, and Dennis, who had become a tower of strength for us, after I explained to PaviElle he was a good nurse and she did not need to be scared of him.

She was still in a coma and there were no male nurses on the sixth floor, so after Maureen and Dennis left, it took five female nurses to put PaviElle in the bed, change her diaper and then put her back in the chair. As I looked on with a deep lump in my throat and a pain in my heart, I realized right then that this part of our journey would be difficult. I got extremely upset when PaviElle pooped and I could not find a nurse fast enough to clean her. I quickly got the basin with water, soap, diaper and cream ready and began to change her myself until a nurse came.

Seeing my sweet daughter sitting in a pile of poo, made me sob hysterically, especially as I knew my skills and strength were not enough to change her by myself. Several nurses came and asked me what happened, but I could barely speak through the tears. When almost too much to bear, but the prayers I just shared helped me to cope with the new intrusion. PaviElle, despite her comatose state seemed more focused and responsive and she continued to sit up in the chair for longer periods of time and doing well with therapy.

July rolled in and the days seemed very busy. One day I stepped out of the room for a moment and when I returned I noticed that they had taken blood from PaviElle's left arm instead of using the PIC Line that was surgically placed in her arm. The PIC line nurse had explained in detail that the line would prevent PaviElle from being stuck constantly when blood needed to be drawn. I was furious with the nurse, who claimed that the use of the line was not ordered, so I then went to the doctor who said it was written in PaviElle's chart.

As soon as I got that sorted out the next hurdle was sodium. Dr. Silver came to inform me that her sodium level was going back up. I explained to her that it had happened in PICU and they had given her water, and her sodium level had then come down. Evidently, the last bottle of water she got was just before she was moved to the sixth floor. I asked Dr. Silver why did she stop getting water and she explained that PaviElle's sodium level had returned to normal. I then asked; if an adult like myself had no water to drink, wouldn't the sodium level go up? She said yes, but PaviElle's formula had water.

I covered my face in frustration and disbelief. Shortly after another doctor came to the room to speak to the medical team that had discussed her sodium problem, and decided PaviElle would begin getting water immediately. The nurse returned with water and that

that the charge nurse rushed in to help me with cleaning her, plus the entire bed linen had to be changed. By this time I was totally drained because I was definitely not impressed with the care my daughter was receiving. All the fears I had developed pertaining to her being transferred to the sixth floor was being realized. Then hooray!!! One of the student doctors came to inform me that her sodium level had gone down because she got the water. But then, to my absolute consternation when Dr. Hernandez and her team came to examine PaviElle she had the audacity to give me information about the hospital's psychology department, advising me to talk with them. Of course, I refused, and told her all I needed was PaviElle to get well, go to rehab and go home. I thought to myself what is a psychologist going to do for me now besides asking me to relate what I was trying so hard to forget. I was sure this was not the appropriate time.

Maureen, my favorite nurse, and Dr. Salano, my favorite doctor, came up from PICU to visit us and see how things were going. That filled my heart with complete joy, knowing they were thinking of our well being and took time out of their hectic schedule to visit.

Another friendly face came to visit in the person of one of the attorneys from Rosen and Rosen the law firm my husband and I had retained for our lawsuit against the Palm Beach County hospital and staff. After I told the attorney about my tragedy, she hugged me and believe it or not, I felt better for that moment. It was late in the afternoon on this particular day and the bed was not yet made. The nurse had several patients, so waiting was now customary. All three therapy specialists, physical, occupational and speech therapists, would have poured water in her glass after she drank her juice. She said sometimes she did, but I told her please do not do that to my daughter. I really became seriously concerned, very worried actually, as to what would happen to my child if I was not always there. However, some of the nurses were great and deserve recognition for their dedication, compassion and hard work. In PICU there was Maureen, Janice, Dennis, Chris and Jade, then on the sixth floor Denise, Doreen, Sharon and Rhonda.

The ratio of nurse to patient was crazy on the sixth floor; therefore it was extremely difficult and almost impossible for any patient to receive quality care. It seemed all the staff was overworked, including the nutritionist Meryl, who finally came to see me to sort out the formula. She promised that she would discuss changing the feed to one that had no milk, less sodium and no corn because PaviElle was not getting enough food. At this time PaviElle was weighing only 76 pounds, and it was unbelievable the fight and struggle I had to go through to see the nutritionists and get them to find a scale to weigh her. I had to fight and basically act like a raving lunatic to get their attention on everything including pointing out that PaviElle was starving, looking like the starving children from famine ravaged parts of Africa that one sees on some television reports. Thank God, every time I protested, I was RIGHT. A prime example of my frustration was the situation with the nurses constantly changing PaviElle's diaper and I kept pointing out something was wrong because of the huge amount and appearance of her poo. I kept being ignored until I screamed in frustration resulting in a doctor coming to investigate, and who after hearing me out ordered a culture to be wanted me to wear the gown and mask and I refused because I told the doctor, if I were not persistent and behave like a raving lunatic, nothing would have been done.

The nights were the usual hell. I had to keep checking PaviElle's diaper and then ask for help to change it. But when I got a little sleep I was constantly awakened by an aide coming in to take vital signs, plus the deafening sound of the feeding machine and the nonstop cry of a sick baby in the next room. As soon as I would change, massage and put PaviElle back to sleep there came the aide to take vitals sign again. I barely got any sleep at nights, and very early in the morning the aide would be there again to take more vitals and blood.

Then there were the huge team of doctors, consultants and experts, who seemed baffled by PaviElle's tragedy. They kept asking me the same question repeatedly: "Why did the nurse at the other hospital give her VERSED? Was she having a procedure? If she had respiratory problems why give her something to further suppress her system?" Each time I had to rehash the events, relating the tragic events, I would break down and sob.

One of the puzzling things at nights was why a simple feeding machine created such a challenge for Nurse Maria. Every time she was on duty and came to feed her it looked like a struggle of great proportions to set the machine. Most of the times I had to help her or another nurse had to come to the rescue.

The mistakes and missteps kept piling up. The nurse comes, draws to the nurse's station and on the top of my voice demand they call the doctor. They tried to make so many excuses why they could not contact the doctor or disturb her unless there was an emergency. The stupid chain of command was for them to speak to the resident, but that doctor could not make a decision. But, I prevailed with them until they finally called PaviElle's doctor, and handed me the telephone. When I explained my concern about the large dosage and medication PaviElle was getting, the doctor immediately agreed with me and spoke to the nurse practitioner who had to apologize to me.

At that juncture I really felt I had my full of all the nonsense, but God stepped in. Someone must have called the head of Patient Relations, because Elizabeth Hollar from that department suddenly appeared in PaviElle's room. She said she was there to talk to me because there seemed to be some concern about my daughter's care. I proceeded to tell her all the good and the bad. I gave accolades and compliments to Maureen and the PICU staff including Dr. Salano, Dennis, Chris and Janice. When Elizabeth asked, me what were some of the things I wanted to improve, I suggested that the nurses should be more consistent in administering medication and that the care they offer would be more effective if they had less patients per nurse, not five patients to one nurse as existed. With tears running down my cheeks I told her it was not humanly possible for any nurse to be effective under those conditions. I explained to her that nurse Maria was taking PaviElle's blood pressure on the same arm with PIC Line and telling me that medication like Reglan can go into the formula. I also told her she was putting medications in the feed and I knew for sure the medication should have gone into the IV.

at nights undisturbed. I had been asking them all along if they ate all day and all night.

Chantal, an African American nurse, the first one I met so far, appeared to be doing things by the orders written in PaviElle's chart. I was extremely grateful, and thanked God, that the staff was finally listening. PaviElle actually slept through the night after these changes were made.

Around this time, Marcella, a great nurse, entered the mix of nurses. She checked every two hours and made sure PaviElle was kept dry, but forgot to put the Cyclosporine in the blood she drew. This was quickly corrected to my great relief.

However, all was still not well. There was this nurse, named Pansy, who came into the room and asked me if I needed help changing my daughter's diaper. I told her she had that wrong, that it was her job to change PaviElle with me assisting her. I complained to the director of nursing, after Pansy persisted to argue with me, telling me it was my job to change my child. I told the director to never again schedule that nurse to care for PaviElle. My request was granted and I was told there were complaints about her by others. There were so many mistakes, nerve racking incidents, shouting, screaming, tears and apologies that occurred at Jackson, it was just unbelievable. I had to fight for everything including whether the formula should be hot or cold, water or no water, wrong doses of medicines, allergic medications, clean the room, toilet paper, blankets, towels, washcloths and clean sheets. There was an evening and entire night

I must be fair and make mention all the nurses who became protectors of PaviElle and provided her with excellent care almost as if they were family. These nurses include Sharon who became Auntie Sharon, Doreen, Chantal, Marcella, Sherry, Rodeline, Reginer, and Joyce who seemed to know how to make PaviElle sleep through the night. Joyce always gave me hope that my daughter would be well again, and told me stories of other patients with similar condition who had bounced back, in an effort to keep me encouraged. I felt so at peace when she was the nurse on duty at nights, especially those rare nights when I had to go home for change of clothes. Nurse Joyce was truly a blessing and source of comfort for both of us.

Reflection of Jackson Memorial's sixth floor.

Of special note is the incident that took place between Dr. Connely, a resident, and I. After speaking with the dietitian and Dr. Hernandez about all the changes that were to be made about the time and temperature of feedings, Dr. Connely was obviously peeved about my queries that were not written in the chart. I stood at the nurse station until she got Dr. Belkine to approve the order, but she refused to call Dr. Hernandez. Then she ordered me to go back to my room because I was disturbing the other patients, or she would call security. I got so mad I told her to go ahead call security. Shouting even louder I told her if I had stood up stronger at the hospital in Palm Beach my child would not be brain damaged. With that she relented, went into her cubbyhole office and called Dr. Hernandez as I had requested, and all was changed because of my persistence.

Another resident doctor wanted to put PaviElle in a cage like structure around the bed and a straight jacket. Trust me; I again lost it when this was suggested. Again, I went to the nurse's station and told the head nurse, Jackie, if anyone tried to restrain my child who had been moving and trying to come out of the coma, I would return with a gun and shoot them all. Jackie looked into my eyes and said, Mrs. McLaughlin no one will restrain PaviElle. Please go home as you planned and get some rest and new clothes."

I told her thanks and was finally convinced to leave without worry. I slept very little and kept calling to make sure my wishes were kept. Surprisingly, the resident who wanted to restrain my child called me to apologize and further discuss my concerns. She agreed that PaviElle was definitely fighting to come out of the coma and should not be restricted. What seemed so shocking to me about this resident was everything she prescribed or every question I had she had to refer to her text book, especially when it related to medications. This made me very frightened and nervous each time she was the doctor on the shift. She appeared so unsure and had no sense of authority or self confidence. Things seemed so great and hopeful some days, while on others everything looked so out of reach and hopeless. One day with PaviElle vomiting, I stood staring through the huge window in her room, feeling broken and deflated. It was frightening to see dark green liquid flying out of her mouth. Everyone panicked as her progress went into reverse. "What now?" I asked the doctors, but no one knew for sure. The vomiting was diagnosed as reflux, caused by the chemo and ridiculous amounts of other medications. A probe was inserted into PaviElle's throat with a pump device from which

She proceeded to give me a long list of all the problems PaviElle had of which I had to remind her that all the bacteria she referred to was contracted in the hospital. She had to come off her high horse with her superior attitude and agreed with me.

Another nightmare manifested itself when PaviElle kept groaning and moaning continuously. I brought it to the attention of the doctors and nurses, but again they tried to convince me there was nothing to worry about. As usual I kept telling them something had to be wrong for her to be moaning constantly and at an increased level. Finally, they decided to humor me and did a cat scan of her kidneys. Sure enough, it was discovered that she had kidney stones for which they wanted to do laparoscopic surgery, but I was not in agreement. Sanity prevailed when the nephrology team came, then the pediatric urologist, who prescribed an alternative method of Tylenol with Codine and saline liquid to attempt to flush out the stones. Dr. Alvarez, the hematologist agreed with me, that surgery would be too aggressive and invasive. We survived one pain-filled ordeal and trauma, only to be faced with another issue. I was so tired of my child suffering; it was exhausting just to watch. Thoughts of guilt began to consume me as I asked myself why had I listened to the rheumatologist. I should have heeded that small voice telling me not to give any more Kineret in spite of his threats. A mother's instinct about her child is never wrong.

After 45 days in Jackson, which I was not counting, because I was too busy extinguishing blazing fires, and preventing them from killing PaviElle, the social worker paid me a visit. She wanted me to

She quickly said, "Oh no; Medicaid will pick up where the insurance company stops, but you have to fill out some forms and go across the street to another building and meet with a specialist."

At that moment, I felt so sick, my stomach felt like it collapsed and I was about to pee and have a bowel movement simultaneously right there in her presence. My brain raced as I thought of other patients who were experiencing a similar fate. I asked myself, "What kind of America is this, with insurance companies telling you on your dying bed, THEY WILL NO LONGER PAY?" This was an experience I have never forgotten, and hope it will not occur again for the remainder of mine or my daughter's life. I also learned that when you are on Medicaid, you are treated only with the cheaper generic drugs. Even when the more expensive drugs will make you better they simply extend the use of the generic drugs. I got so angry about this when the CDIF she contracted in the hospital would not get better and they insisted on giving her the generic drug. I asked the doctor who explained that Medicaid would not pay for the brand name drug even though it would cure the condition faster. My rage after hearing this is impossible to explain so I persisted until they changed the medication which took care of the bacteria.

The next battle was trying to move PaviElle to the hospital's in-house rehabilitation unit which by all accounts and research is supposed to be excellent. I had countless meetings with the head-nurse and the rehab doctor, Dr. Restrepo, who seemed very charming and agreed with me that PaviElle would be a good candidate after he examined her and looked at the medications she was taking.

The incident that really made me know PaviElle was totally aware of what was going on around her was actually quite funny. The neurologist who came to visit her once, when we just arrived at Jackson, barely did anything but prescribed Baklophen to relax her muscles. When I did my research I discovered one of the side effects of this drug was drowsiness. So I kept trying to figure out if she was sleeping all the time, how would she be able to get her physical, occupational and speech therapies. I had explained to the neurology nurse that the dosage was too strong for PaviElle, but she kept disagreeing, until I was proven right again. I consistently told these doctors that my child was not like all children and was extremely sensitive to drugs. Maybe now they would believe me.

When we were ready to go to rehab, Dr. Lopeda the neurologist came to do his final examination. He never came back since his first visit but would only send his nurse. I always asked her for the doctor and she would explain that he is extremely busy and she was his representative. I would always ask her, how could Dr.Lopeda keep prescribing medication for my daughter and never come to see her? As he tried to examine PaviElle she pulled her foot out of his hand and kicked him, with a force I had never seen. I assumed she was mad because they would not listen to my concerns about the medications and he never came to examine her or follow her progress.

In mid-July PaviElle had a seizure. Panic ensued and an army of doctors descended on us. This was another delay in our going to rehab. The prescription was for a nurse or aide to sit in the room all night and all day in case another seizure happened. Also Xeoponex and also ordered Triliptol to prevent seizures. Every medication they prescribed for her, she would display all or some of the side effects. They seemed to have a drug for everything, but not for healing and recovery of the brain.

Once we survived all this, Dr. Stricker, the orthopedic surgeon, came to see if PaviElle could stand. He said she could, but her second toe was the most injured and would need to be amputated. I told him God's miracle would continue to heal her toes so there would be no amputation. I guess he did not consult with the plastic surgery team because I already told them, absolutely NO SURGERY on her toes.

The delay in PaviElle's recovery kept me apprehensive, but I could not allow myself to stop celebrating the small miracles every day. As soon as I got a victory or two, there would be some unbelievable event that arose. This required me to fight, get enraged, and scream at the top of my lungs until someone responded. I had to come to terms with the set- backs, delays and various treatments that PaviElle had to have and complete before she could go to the rehab unit and closer to going home. I kept rallying for the therapies to continue, so visible progress could be made and they did. I counted down the weeks of chemo treatments, EEG, echo-cardiogram and other tests she had to endure. Most nights as I laid on my makeshift bed made from the huge chair in the room, piling it with numerous blankets and sheets to create some sense of softness and comfort, I realized you don't need much to survive in life. I prayed constantly and kept thanking God for all the small improvements I witnessed in PaviElle that day.

not go down. I felt like I could not eat because my child could not eat or drink. The cleaning lady would read the sign I had placed above PaviElle's head every day. It read, "PAVIELLE is TOTALLY HEALED in the NAME of JESUS" Then she would share her own tragedies and triumphs and when toilet paper, blankets and sheets were scarce she made sure I got what I needed. I began to get massage oils, movies and whatever I requested from the recreation department. A young lady, who showed such empathy and care for the tragedy we had experienced kept making several suggestions that would make PaviElle more comfortable.

PaviElle grinding her teeth was another hurdle to jump. As usual, no one was concerned but me and the solution was simple, a mouth guard placed over her teeth. It helped the grinding and the biting of

All the nurses ignored her dental hygiene, because they were afraid that PaviElle would bite them when they tried to brush her teeth. I had to take that job because I was determined that her beautiful teeth that I had so diligently taken care of was not going down the drain. I went to the store and bought a tongue cleaner and brush, then went to work to eliminate the odor and clean her teeth.

Oh how wonderful it was to see how she cooperated with me each day and night, as I gently cleaned her tongue and brushed her teeth, and reminding her how beautiful they were, and the compliments she always received from everyone in the past because of her gorgeous and captivating smile.

was also a nurse. She told me all the great success of the unit and of all the celebrities like Christopher Reeves who were treated there with great improvement. I was, however, not impressed with the way the unit looked old and in need of updating, repair and decorating. It seemed dingy, dark and depressing for a place of recovery. I politely smiled and made it appear that I was in agreement with all she was saying, but the honesty in me made me ask her why the place looked so old and dark. To my surprise she explained that they should have gone through a major renovation but had experienced numerous delays. She tried to convince me to look past the appearance of the place because the nursing care was excellent and the therapy was intense and exceptional. Her words sank in and I felt great relief that my instincts were right.

Before we could go to rehab the NG tube for feeding had to be surgically placed in PaviElle's stomach, to replace the one in her nose. I got the rare choice of choosing the appropriate one for her and it was done. Then there was the cleaning, and instructions for the tube, which felt very overwhelming at the time, but became easy after a few times doing the task.

But there was another challenge before PaviElle was transferred to rehab when she was soaked from head to toe in her own urine because the hospital had no linen due to a major problem with the contractor who did the laundry. This incident threw me into a state of depression and deep sadness with a feeling of helplessness. I thought to myself the numerous sets of linens I owned between me and my mother and here we are with none available to use in this

Chapter 6

od was about to make a big move. He sent a team of angels, headed by Prophetess Dr. Charmaine Peart, to pay us a visit.

I previously made contact with her after several calls and messages left on her cell and home phone. Her number was given to me by my aunt who had heard her speak in Baltimore at a women's conference, and asked her to come see us in the hospital. Several people had come to pray with us, but somehow this felt different. I felt Prophetess and her prayer team were being sent specially by God himself. When Dr. Peart called she gave me a date and time that she and her team could come. She asked for the room number and I told her we were on the sixth floor but advised her to follow the sound of the screaming and moaning and that would be PaviElle's room.

They arrived early in the evening on Tuesday July 17, 2007. As they entered the door I immediately felt like a magnet was pulling Prophetess towards me and without any introduction I knew she was the person I had spoken to on the telephone. She introduced everyone else on the prayer team – Bishop Gayle her brother, Sisters Novelette and Madge, and Brother Campbell. She also noticed the sign I had placed over PaviElle's head that read "PaviElle is Totally experienced in PICU when Claudina prayed, but this felt somehow bigger. Before they left Prophetess instructed me to anoint PaviElle with the remaining olive oil they had brought for seven days and call her when I was finished doing so. She told me this with assurance in her voice that a miracle would take place after the seventh day of anointing. No one knew what God would do and how huge it was going to be, but my expectation and belief were off the charts.

Maureen, Dr. Selana, Dr. Nunez all kept visiting and checking PaviElle's progress. They were more surprised and pleased each time they came but insisted that it was because of my love and care for her that made her survive such a tragic and traumatic experience. However, I humbly gave God the glory every time.

I routinely anointed PaviElle exactly the way and at the time I was instructed by Prophetess. The great news came when all the results of each test came back good. My heart was filled, with nothing but HOPE, BELIEVE and TRUST in God and his Goodness.

But there would be several other mistakes made before our sixth floor departure. These included the respiratory therapist giving her a treatment of Albuterol after I told him it had been discontinued by the doctor because of the good results of the tests given to PaviElle. There was also the SMA diagnosis, and the incorrect placement of the feeding tube in her nose, which made the doctor so mad he pulled it out and replaced it himself. Then Ronald McDonald House called the social worker, Bridgette, to say we were no longer in the hospital. I went over to the house to see what was going on only to

McDonald House, a well known charity created to help families in desperate need, when they were at the hospital caring for their children. The female supervisor, who barely spoke any English had nothing much to say, even as her daughter tried to be the translator. Walking back to the hospital I just wept.

Returning to the room gave me no solace because the various diagnosis and missteps kept coming. I consoled myself with the prayer of Prophetess and the prayer team telling myself the miracle would come.

Dr. Podda, my favorite Italian doctor was the attendee for the weekend and he was about to make changes and shake things up, and make me hopeful again. He made radical changes that I had been fighting like changing the feeding schedule, reviewing all medications and discontinuing most of them including Reglan. He ordered plastic surgery to debris the wound under PaviElle's arm from the biopsy that had been done the second day after she was admitted to Jackson, and disconnected the NG tube suction. I was so elated I felt like hugging him and crying with happiness.

After that, I still had to stop a nurse from giving PaviElle some of the medications that were stopped by Dr. Podda. It was now crystal clear to me that if I was not at the hospital everyday my child would have died. I thought of all the families who could not be at the hospital with their loved ones around the clock. What kind of care were their loved ones receiving? This was, and is, insanity.

if the speech therapist could proceed with trying to feed her by mouth. She was resistant to the test and refused to corporate until I coaxed her with a mom's persuasion. We got a big boost when all the therapists agreed that PaviElle would be an excellent candidate for the rehab unit at Jackson because her progress was moving at an unbelievable and miraculous pace.

Dr. Calooze was the outstanding hyperbaric-chamber expert at Jackson MH so I made a request to meet with him. When I did, he recommended a colleague, Dr. Lucy Cohen at Health South Rehab in Sunrise, South Florida, whose work and success with brain injured patients he believed in. To this day I have never met Dr. Cohen because as much effort as I put into calling, and speaking to her staff, the great disappointment was that Health South did not accept Medicaid.

I kept hoping that PaviElle would start eating in very small amounts before we went to rehab but that was not to be. Eating would be delayed until we got home. Dr. Alvarez decided at this point to increase the feed formula because I was concerned that she was suffering from malnutrition.

In preparation for rehab I was briefed about every possible procedure, medication, the PEG tube, which they made seem so difficult, and the situations to expect before we got to rehab. Information overload was my plight but since I wanted her to be moved so badly, I sucked it all in, some things I wrote down but mostly retained everything in my memory. There was more chemotherapy VC16 treatment before

PaviElle would be healed fully in the name and blood of Jesus. I kept wondering what other circumstance the sixth floor staff would create to delay our transfer to rehab. Everyday there was another excuse and more hurdles to jump over. I thought the day might never come.

The final problem that arose was that the rehab staff had to wait for another patient to be discharged so there would be a bed and room available for us. However, the day, a Friday, arrived and Dr. Restrepo and his nurse, Suzie, came to evaluate PaviElle one last time. After the examination of moving and prodding he announced the plan. PaviElle would go to rehab on Monday on a two week trial and her progress would be assessed. If she progressed, the therapy would continue because then the insurance would continue to pay the hospital, but if not she would be sent home, and follow up with outpatient and/or home visits. He said the insurance companies considered rehab a luxury. Needless to say I was shocked on hearing this. Suzie advised me to leave the PIC line, used for drawing blood and give medicine, just in case the various team of doctors she had on the sixth floor followed her to rehab.

The weekend felt like it would never end. All I could think about was the success that PaviElle would have when she began to have all her therapies all day, six days a week for two weeks. Added were classes for her to learn to read, write, do math and relearn Spanish. She was like being a baby once more. But, my joy came and then came crashing down when Monday came and went, and we are still on the sixth floor. I felt myself becoming depressed, so I called Prophetess and told her about my disappointment. She prayed with me and told humor and telling stories about the success of the rehab unit. He said he had good news and bad news, then asked which one I wanted first. I opted for the good news first. He stated that the insurance company would pay for the cost of the rehab, but the bad news was that they would only pay for one week instead of the two weeks he had indicated PaviElle would have been in rehab. I had no choice because I didn't have the financial resources, to pay for the other week, so the insurance company had the final word. How dare they play God with my only child's life? What a healthcare system in the most powerful industrialized nation in the world! I was filled with disbelief and frustration but there was no time to take on that problem. I had to work with what I had been given.

The going to rehab saga continued in a way that was unbelievable. I was the only one who felt a sense of urgency. Everyone was saying tomorrow, and tomorrow wasn't coming fast enough for me. They continued to order more and more test for the reflux disease, CDIF bacteria. August 7, 2007 was the final day for the biggest treatment, Chemo VP16. Remember, it had the power to cure the JRA that was PaviElle's first diagnosis. The list of drugs was absolutely frightening for me so I will list them. Reglan, Flagil, Cyclosporine, Dexamethasone, Norvast, Triliptol, Baclofin, Diflucan, Magnesium, Miralax, Benadryl ,Pentamadine, IBIG and many more.

The medication that brought me face to face with Dr. Fernandez was Vancomycin. When she prescribed it, I asked her what were the side effects. She hesitated, and then said, none really, but a rare one was called Redmans Syndrome. I told her PaviElle was so allergic to drugs came to install and remove the probe that was used to test for Reflux. When she removed it and gave the good news that the result was negative, she hugged and cried with me. Following this good news I was faced with PaviElle having two bowel movements in a row and I kept ringing the bell for help but no one came. She was scheduled and had to go to the operating room for the procedure, to put the G Tube in her stomach but she was still lying in her pooh. The PIC Line nurse had to help me clean her up, only to have her pooh again. When we got to the operating room all the nurses saw my distress and tears, so they quickly pulled her in the room and cleaned her and told me not to worry they would take good care of her.

Dr. Narez from PICU was part of the team that did the surgery for the G Tube and Dr. Abrahams asked if they could do another lumbar puncture to check her bone marrow. I called Lloyd for support in making this decision and we agreed to give permission. PaviElle went to sleep as soon as they gave her a small dose of Propofol. All my memories of the Versed given to her by the nurse of death came rushing back to my mind. I was crying and shaking hysterically. Dr. Narez had to take me to the side and explained that the Propofol was very strong but does not last long so she would be awake quickly. They then wanted to give her morphine for pain but I refused and they gave another drug in the Motrin family. I was on pins and needles until PaviElle woke up which was quick as the doctor had promised. The tube was placed successful and the lumbar puncture showed normalcy. Dr. Hernandez, Dr. Jenifer Garcia and Celine came and assured me that all was well and I should not worry.

needed help, so I rang the bell five times and no one came. It was obvious they were short staffed, because a few nurses had the Flu. Nurse Susanna, the big bad substitute came after the fifth ring of the bell. She stood in the door way with her hands on her hips, furious that I rang the bell so many times. She told me with an authoritative tone of voice that it was my duty to clean PaviElle. I got so mad; I chased her out of the room, went to the nurse's station and told them, "Do not let that bitch come back into my daughter's room again."

I then went to make a formal complaint to Karen who was there for Maureen. I also called Celine to see if she could help expedite a more urgent move to the rehab unit before I lost my mind completely. She called and things began jumping.

It was now August 13, 2007 and I was so stressed because my hope was that was the day to go to rehab. Dr. Solar came to see PaviElle but I noticed she had a cold so I told her she could not come in and she said that was the reason she was wearing a mask. I told her and Nurse Derwin who was also sick, that I could not take the risk of PaviElle getting a virus thus risking another delay in going to rehab. They understood and so I prayed to God and asked him to help us leave the sixth floor before she contracted some virus or bacteria.

When I asked to speak to the rehab nurse, Suzie, I was told she was on vacation. I felt my stomach drop to the floor because no one knew what the hell was going on. My frustration only escalated. That night only made things worse. I bathed PaviElle all by myself, then cautious with her. She shared with me, she had her own troubles then spent time cleaning the G tube and telling me how messy it was. As she continued I felt bad for her and told her my frustration after hearing during the day from Bridgette the social worker that they were still waiting for authorization for PaviElle to go to Rehab.

In the midst of those dark feelings God made something remarkable happen. PaviElle was very restless and barely slept all night but kept saying, while she moaned, "Maaama, maama." Instantly, I began to pray, asking God for patience and forgiveness. On August 15, 2007 as I did my usual stare through the huge window in the hospital room I heard someone say, "You are going to rehab today." Those were the sweetest words I had heard in a very long time. I was filled with exhilaration, joy, thankfulness, appreciation and nervousness all at the same time. I really was not sure what lay ahead, but I was READY for whatever challenges that would come. I packed all PaviElle's and my belongings and was rearing to go. The nurses made sure I had all the supplies they thought might be in short supply at the rehab unit. They were all so happy for me and agreed that she would make great progress in rehab.

It was not until 4:50 p.m. that day that we are permitted to leave. PaviElle was on the gurney and we went rolling down the hallway of the sixth floor to the patient elevator, the one that we took many times for surgery and various tests, but this time it was for the beginning of another chapter. As I began to walk to the elevator I felt someone's arm around my waist. Looking around, I realized it was a woman who worked at the nurse's station who barely spoke to me. She was she squeezed my hand tightly. I began thinking and telling myself never to judge those around you who may seem quiet and show no emotion because they might be the one to observe everything and give you the most profound words of encouragement when you need it most.

Chapter 7

ehabilitation Unit here we come," I said to myself. When we got to the room my heart sank because it was dark and dingy just as I remembered when I took the tour. The bathroom for me was unusable; there was no shower just a toilet and sink. I was forced to wash myself twice a day in a basin I carried with me.

Again, this seeming inconvenience made me realize we needed very little to survive, and material things were not that important in the big scheme of life, especially in the circumstances that had become PavieElle's and my tragedy and devastation. I consoled myself to always be thankful and God will take care of us as He promised in

It was 1:15 a.m. as I laid on the hard chair I managed to get earlier, and made it as comfortable as possible with several blankets and sheets, a routine I had grown accustomed to. The light over PaviElle's head kept flickering, so I got up and went to the nurse's station to ask the nurse on duty if someone from the maintenance department could come and fix it. She said she would call them and someone should be there shortly.

to fix the light myself. While I was on the chair I heard a voice say, "Mommy you're crazy, you're so funny."

Shocked, I fell off the chair and almost broke my leg because it was PaviElle's voice. She had spoken a complete sentence. I began to shout, "Thank you God. Thank you God."

I kissed and hugged her, rubbing her bald head. The nurses hearing the commotion came running to the room asking, "What's wrong, what's wrong?"

I was speechless. I gathered myself and wiped the tears of joy as they ran down my cheeks, but I managed to say, "PaviElle spoke. It is God's miracle."

They began to celebrate with me. One of the nurse's called the doctor on duty. When he came, he tried to hold PaviElle's hand and examine her, but she pulled her hand away from the doctor and screamed "Get away from me, don't touch me."

A short while later I called Lloyd and gave him the great news. I said, "Good morning, are you on your to way to the hospital?"

"No," he replied, but as I held the phone close to PaviElle, she overheard her father's voice, took the phone from me and said, "Right, no Daddy."

"What! Is that PaviElle. She's speaking. Thank God. Thank God. It's the world was heard by God and the process of restoration and healing had finally begun. Marcella, Joyce and Verne from the sixth floor came to visit soon after. They were overjoyed and filled with hope for PaviElle being able to speak again. They were in shock that all this happened on her first night in rehab. Dr. Alvarez also visited and expressed her feelings of happiness for us.

PaviElle had her first sessions of occupational, physical and speech therapy in the rehab unit, soon after this joyful occasion. She tried very hard in therapy and did her best. You could tell she was ready to be finished and go home. Later that afternoon, in an attempt to test her memory, I asked her if she wanted Dunkin Donuts, and she said "Yes."

It was obvious that she did remember our visit to get donuts before she was stricken ill. I then said, "You have to swallow all the time, so the speech therapist can give us the okay for you to eat."

"All rightie," she replied.

These were words she liked using before she was stricken, so I knew for sure her memory was returning. I called my aunt to let PaviElle speak to her. My aunt asked her if she wanted chicken, her favorite meat and she answered, "Yea, yea."

After my aunt hung up, I asked PaviElle if she was cold, and she said, "No, not really." Turning to the television set which was on; I asked her, "Do you want me to switch the channel?"

He then asked, "Do you want to watch television?"

"Yea," she said.

"Do you want to watch the Disney channel?"

"Yea," she again replied.

"Or do you want me to change the channel to the Spanish station?" This had been one of her favorite channels in the past.

"Yea," she replied.

"Do you remember your Spanish?" I asked.

"Yes," she said.

The phone rang again, and it was another of my aunts, having heard the good news that PaviElle was talking; calling to speak to her. When I handed her the phone to listen she immediately recognized my aunt's voice and said, "Hi Auntie Fay."

After this phone call I asked her if she wanted to speak to her grandmother, my mom, and she said yes. Of course my mom was ecstatic, in a state of shock really, and kept repeating, "Oh Pavi, oh Pavi."

It was now 6:29 p.m. and I pressed the button for the nurse. Just as

"Can Mommy have some then?' the nurse asked.

"No," she said again, "It's mine, it's all mine".

Hearing her speak and seeing her interaction with the nurse I felt so gratified, so full of praise for God, all the love for her multiplied several times over in my heart, and I said, "I love you so much, little

"I love you, too," she replied.

It was now 7:00 p.m. and I told her to say thank you Jesus and she said "Thank, you God, praise God'"

An hour or so later and I felt a little tired, so I told PaviElle I would get the nurse to change her diaper, and she replied, "I don't care mommy. I love you."

Early in the morning, I got up to change her, and she said,
"I love you Mommy, you are so funny."

Everyone wanted to hear her speak so they kept telling me to keep her talking and ask lots of questions. I kept her talking. When the nurse came to attend to her she told her, "Get away from me woman."

This made the nurse laugh, telling her, "As long as you are talking, all is good."

Then, Kassi, another nurse came to give her water and she resisted. I had to tell PaviElle the nurse was a nice person, to which she replied, "Yea, right."

Later meeting with the physical therapist she said, "My name is PaviElle."

When Maria, the teacher, asked her to spell her name and the word, cat, she replied, "I'm not retarded."

When Maria asked her if she wanted to go home, she said, "Yes."

During, the physical therapy session Maria returned to the room and PaviElle told her, "Get the hell away from me woman."

I took her back to her room and she said to me, "Put it there," and I asked put what? She said, "The food," referring to food on a tray that had been brought in for me.

I reminded her she could not eat yet but she could take a sip of juice with the straw just like in speech therapy.

I called my mom to tell her about the day and PaviElle kept saying, "I don't want to be here."

When I got off the phone, she said, "I want to read to you mom."

She pointed to a book and asked me to read for her. Soon after, she

Lloyd asked her how she was doing and she replied, "Fine," her favorite response.

When she was off the phone I told her I had to clear her nose and she asked me if her ears were dirty too. I reminded her that I cleaned them yesterday. When I read for her the story spoke about dreams and I asked PaviElle what are her dreams. She said "I have lots of

I told her to say "Winter Moon Family," the title of the book, and she repeated this clearly. I asked her if she had poo in her pants, and she replied, "No man."

I put my nose close to her to smell if she did and she said, "I'm fine."

At 3:05 p.m. she announced, "I'm hungry."

I told her again she had to be able to swallow first. I asked her to repeat what I said and she said "Swallow, swallow, swallow." I read another story about a woman who had seven children and she said, "That's a lot of kids."

I then challenged her to say 'proposition' and she easily said the word. She kept doing her lips a strange way I asked why she was doing that, and she said, "I have no idea."

The story I was reading to her mentioned fifty bond fires and she said, "Oh wow!"

She replied without hesitation, "My house is at 245 Westwood Circle East." I was elated and filled with hope, as the tears filled my eyes and came streaming down my face.

August 18, was yet another great day in her recovery. She began to sing her favorite song by the singer Usher, called "Confessions." Maria was shocked. After physical therapy with Maria went very well, I asked PaviElle if she wanted to go outside and she said, "Yes."

This was the first time she would be seeing the outdoors since she was admitted to the hospital in Palm Beach County on May 2, when the nightmare began. When she saw the food that was brought in for me she reached for the eggs. I again reminded her that Jenny, the speech therapist would have to clear her to eat before she could swallow. PaviElle said, "Bring her right now, right now."

While we were outside you could see the smile and joy in her face, especially when she had a visit from some of the good nurses from the sixth floor. Ms. Joyce, Marcella, Renae, Sharon, Chantal and Kina. PaviElle had her first shower also on this day and she was very scared of the water, but it went well. The shower was given to her by my cousin Sandra who was so faithful in visiting us at the hospital as often as she could. Her strength that day showed me how much she cared.

I had to go home for clothes because I had only a few items and kept wearing them over and over. This was the first time I was leaving her since we got to rehab. I was very concerned and had a nervous words to me, "Don't look at the place, results are good and the nursing care is excellent."

When I saw her enter the room and said she would be PaviElle's nurse for the evening and until 7:00 a.m. Sunday, I said to her, "Praise the Lord, I can go home tonight."

She replied, "Go ahead, don't worry. There is also another wonderful nurse, Mr. Charles, working with me tonight. He just returned from vacation in Jamaica."

In my heart I thanked God for His blessing, with my eyes filled with tears. When Lloyd came that evening, we were excited to update him, on all the wonderful things we experienced, that day, and we left for home. Of course, when I got home, I called the nurse's station in the rehab unit to check on the situation, but they assured me PaviElle was fine, and asked if I wanted to speak with her on the telephone. I quickly said yes. It was so exciting to hear my daughter's sweet voice on the telephone. This was something I had so longed for, because before she was sick she would call me every day on her phone as soon as she got out of classes, and in her sweet girlish voice ask me where I was parked so she could get to me quickly. I heard that girlish voice again as we spoke, and I felt a feeling that can never be explained.

She and I went outdoor again the next day, but she got a fever that night. The nurse gave her Tylenol and I placed cold rags on her forehead, something I saw done while she was in PICU and the sixth so well so fast. They encouraged me to keep going but to take care of myself and try to eat because I was losing so much weight. God was obviously sustaining me and I kept remembering my mother's words, "You are strongest at your weakest point."

Dr. Restrepo the rehab doctor was away for a few days and Susie the nurse practitioner was on vacation during our first days in the unit. When they returned and saw all the progress PaviElle had made they could not believe their eyes and ears. Dr. Restrepo kept saying "Neuroplasticity" over and over. I asked what it meant and he explained that when someone suffers a brain injury, when they changed location with input from a new environment, this is sometimes the result. He kept pacing around the room as if he was puzzled, and I kept telling him, "I told you she needed to come to rehab a long time ago because that was what my spirit was telling me".

Dr. Restrepo was one of the doctors who always read the sign I had placed over PaviElle's bed on the sixth floor, that read "PaviElle is Totally Healed in the Name of Jesus." He would support my belief, that she would be healed and restored. I always thanked him for acknowledging the sign each time he came to the room.

She continued to do very well in all her therapies, but Joney and the other speech therapist, along with Dr. Maroon got mad with me because I tried to feed PaviElle with a straw, to drink some apple juice that she asked for. This is something I always did, especially on the days when she had only one session of any therapy because session, so they came to me and asked for my help to make her swallow. I flatly refused, telling them they treated me like a criminal the day before, so how could they now need my help.

Although PaviElle was very ill she knew and heard everything, then reacted fiercely with anyone who was rude, abusive and did not listen to me. It was simply amazing to watch.

On August 20, the Miami-Dade County School representative came to give me forms, for her to attend school in the rehab unit. She asked a lot of questions, which I answered but I was still reeling with disgust over the incident with the speech therapists. The lady left a stack of forms for me to fill out and Dr. Restrepo to sign. I was not in any mood or frame of mind to fill out the forms, so I tackled them the following day and returned them to her. After she left I decided to check PaviElle's diaper. To my joy she helped me lift herself out of the wheel chair and also to get back into the chair to sit. Immediately my heart was healed and I truly felt she did it because she knew I was mad and wanted to do something to please me, and make me happy and hopeful again. She definitely succeeded.

It was now time to remove the PIC Line because the doctor suspected it was the source of an infection that she had contracted. The PIC Line did not grow any bacteria, the doctor explained so they took blood, to do a CBC and Culture, because her white blood cell count, was going up.

PaviElle was very uncooperative in all therapies the next day. I thought rebellion and did not want to cooperate with anything and anyone, but me. They all agreed and all discussions were done away from her room.

Doreen and Sharon, two of PaviElle's favorite nurses came to visit during that time and cheered both of us up. While they were there, the recreational therapist, who obviously was told about the incidents and PaviElle's mood, came bearing gifts and several other items for her to choose from.

As she played a Disney CD PaviElle began to sing along with the songs and Doreen and Sharon were excited and over joyed. Dr. Hernandez from GI also came and I took the opportunity to ask about increasing the feed formula because she was not gaining any weight. She told me she would send her GI team to see her to evaluate increasing the formula. I was very thankful.

Dr. Restrepo and Suzie were so excited about PaviElle's rapid recovery in the first week of rehab that they became impatient and wanted to make the process move faster. They came in for their morning meeting with me and asked me to think about giving her Ritalin or Amantadine. Both medications they explained would accelerate the speed of her already fast-pace restoration. They did not want an immediate answer, but asked me to do the research and get back to them that afternoon. I quickly called my cousin Simone in New York, explained to her what was asked of me, and asked her to research both drugs. As she read the side effects of the drugs my heart raced with anxiety, nervousness and disbelief. I then called Dr. Rubin my

Later that afternoon when they returned for an answer I told them my answer was absolutely no. No Ritalin and no Amantadine, and that I would continue to wait on God's timing. I then asked them to consider what I thought would be a better and sure thing to speed up PaviElle's recovery. With keen attention they listened to my request. It was simple. I requested a pass for Saturday to take her home to her familiar surroundings. That I said would be the best medicine for her. They asked me to give them time to discuss my request with the team and promised to get back to me.

While I waited for the answer a few scary things happened, that might have delayed getting the pass to go home for the day. PaviElle's blood test showed some bacteria and they wanted to give her Vancomiacin, the same medication she had such a violent reaction to before. I said I was not in agreement to her being given that drug and asked Dr. Mareno to page Dr. Alvarez who agreed with Dr. Abraham to go back into PaviElle's file. Dr. Duncan, who was on call came later to tell me they would use Cephapine, an antibiotic she took already, but just to be safe, they would give her Benadryl first. Things were beginning to test my patience again but PaviElle continued to show progress in all therapies. Maria put her in a new garment that helped her to sit up straight. It looked like a diving suit, only it was in several pieces, with bright cobalt blue and more complicated to put on the body.

The formula issue was not addressed by the GI. The wound specialist who I kept asking for but who never came, finally showed up with no solution or new ointment for PaviElle's major sores, especially her toes. I kept complaining to Eddie from maintenance that the wheel calories, but not protein, to her diet. The multivitamins, vitamin C and yogurt I had discussed with Dr. Duncan, also began.

I was being forced into in a situation to completely lose my temper and use my loudest voice to get results. The cleaning lady kept coming everyday but I noticed the spilled milk was still on the floor each time we returned to the room after therapy. I decided to clean the floor myself and was shocked at not only the spilt milk, but the amount of dirt I was seeing on the bleach cloth I was using. I made a decision to save all the bleach cloths that I used to show the big wigs, after I showed it to Jillian and told my friend Dr. Rubin on the phone. I demanded to see the head of house cleaning to show her the bleach cloths I had used to clean the floor. When she came and saw how filthy the clothes were she immediately called someone on the phone and there was action. The cleaning crew that came removed every piece of furniture including the bed and all other items from the room in my presence. By the time we returned from therapy, the room was so clean, you could literally see your face through the shine on the floor. We had the cleanest room in the entire rehab unit. All the staff and nurses began to congratulate me and the word began to spread, about my accomplishment with the cleaning head-huncho.

Good news followed as Dr. Mareno came to say the blood culture result was negative, but the antibiotic would continue until Saturday, the day I was expecting to be able to go home for the day. Needless to say I was mad because Dr. Duncan had clearly stated that if the blood culture was negative, the Cephatine would stop immediately.

day before we would be able to go home for a day. Dr. Karana was covering for Dr. Restrepo for two days but he gave the approval for us to get the one day pass.

Although I was totally wiped out and exhausted, I looked forward to going home the next day with PaviElle so she could see her house and room for the first time in nearly four months. Sharon, Chantal, Jennifer and Dr. Podia all came to visit that night. Marla, the dietitian came to see if the weight she got was accurate or were there any changes since the Lipids were added to the feed formula. Dr. Striker the orthopedic surgeon also came and ordered that PaviElle must wear the sandals he had prescribed, but which she hated, during physical therapy, especially while standing exercises were done. The GI team did their rounds to check on the G Tube and said everything looked good but gave specific orders, that the area must only be taped during therapy and removed promptly afterwards.

I took PaviElle to the sixth floor for a visit. All the nurses and staff were so excited to see her and the progress she made. It was now breaking my heart because as she got better she began crying real tears and saying "I am hungry, mom." Rosie the nurse tried talking to her with no success, she said a lollipop might do the trick. I told her I was willing to try anything to stop her from crying. The lollipop worked for a bit but the frothing of her mouth continued. All this was frustrating and annoying, but I told myself patience and time was the only hope.

The next day, August 25, the sun shun brightly from a very clear, blue appetite for. When Lloyd came to the hospital that morning to pick us up, she was so excited, I had to remind her it was only for the day and we had to return at 8:00 p.m. otherwise she would lose her benefits and the insurance would no longer pay for the rehab room and therapy. She was clearly disappointed but understood.

We had to do only physical therapy that glorious morning, which I had scheduled for the first and earliest appointment. The PT had to be there, to show Lloyd and I, how to get PaviElle in and out of the car and the wheel chair. That exercise went well and we were on our wonderful journey to home sweet home. She had to sit in the front passenger seat of the car because it was easier to get in and out, without possible incident. We also had to pad the seat to prevent any bodily accident, however she did great.

PaviElle reacted to being in her room immediately. She laid in her bed in her usual position and did not want to get out. She asked her dad to take her in the wheelchair to each room of the house, then Lloyd lifted her out of the wheelchair and she sat down in her favorite chair, beside the sliding glass door.

Then she had guests. Dr. Rubin arrived first and then my friend, Joan. She was so excited to see them. We all had such a great day and it got even better, when PaviElle said she wanted to pee. Joan being the nurse, rolled the wheelchair into her bathroom, placed her on the toilet and she peed. We all celebrated the moment because this was something they had tried so many times at the hospital and she refused to even try. When everyone left it was almost time to return

I explained to her, that she had to go back to rehab. She replied, "Who cares," and told Lloyd "Daddy I can walk on my feet okay."

The ride back to the hospital was solemn, and quiet. I announced to Lloyd that this would be the last weekend we would be driving back to Jackson Memorial Hospital. He looked at me with concern in his eyes and asked, "Who will take care of her when you bring her

l replied "Me".

He was obviously stunned. He reminded me that I would not be able to do it on my own, and he had to go to work. I said, "Don't worry

To be truthful, all I had was my resolve that PaviElle needed to be home to recover, no matter how difficult and impossible it seemed then. I had complete faith and trust that God would help me get through and give me the strength and knowledge I would need.

When we returned to the hospital, PaviElle instantly asked her dad to take her to the room. She seemed depressed, very reserved and quiet, while I was telling the nurses all the success we had at home. Joyce and Denise came to visit and Lloyd left for the journey back home. My report was obviously noted because on Monday Dr. Restrepo and Suzie came to say they heard the good report and would have a meeting with the entire team, including me, to make a decision about when PaviElle could go home for good. He explained

Deadly Negligence

someone had to be at my house to receive all these things prior to setting the exit date.

I went on rapid speed to get everything done. The most difficult form to sign was the one for the disabled parking. When the administrator said she would check the box for permanent disability she noticed my tears and distress and stopped to console me, saying she was doing this to save me the aggravation of having to repeat the process if she did not walk again. I rejected that thought and continued to cry, while quietly telling God PaviElle must walk again.

She did very well in therapy the day after she had visited her home, and it is clear that the day at home had been good for her. After all the therapies that day I was told the conference to discuss PaviElle's chances of going home would be at 2:00 p.m. I was happy that the process for my child to go home was about to begin. As I reflected on this positive development I saw another mom in the hallway crying. Her daughter, Chandra was regressing, but had begun to walk. I told her to thank God that she was walking and she should continue to pray.

When I entered the conference room for the meeting I saw it was full with all the experts seated, with one chair empty for me to sit in. I felt a little intimidated but put forth a very confident face, ready for the decision I wanted for my daughter. The decision for us to go home was made after a long discussion, with everyone giving their opinions. I listened but asked no questions because I only wanted one answer. Then, at last, Dr. Restrepo made the announcement I

Walking back to the room to tell PaviElle the good news, I felt like I had just won the lottery. When I told PaviElle she exclaimed, "Yea! We are going home!"

I changed her poo diaper and she hugged me, and then said, "1-2-3 back in the chair." She was starting to use her left hand and I was glad. I called Lloyd to share the great news. It was coming through the phone line that he was nervous, but happy at the same time.

On Tuesday morning we were still celebrating the good news of going home. She was doing the therapy with great passion and a determination no one could explain. She kept telling everyone she encountered, "I am going home tomorrow."

She was also happy to tell Dr. Mareno she was going home. Dr. Mareno gave us our final instructions, which included returning to see Dr. Podda the first or second Monday, or Tuesday, in September. She gave us the good news that PaviEllle's white blood cell count was down from 30,000 to 20,000.

Maureen, my favorite nurse from PICU came to visit and wished us good luck for going home but she had some fantastic news herself. She had been promoted to a nurse practitioner. I had always told her she should be a doctor because she was so smart and had such knowledge. She shared that she was studying to take the medical exams and without doubt I told her she would definitely pass. I was so happy for her because she needed to spread her wings and share her expertise. Every patient and their family should have an encounter

Deadly Negligence

a visit before we left the hospital. His support from the first week we got to Jackson was unwavering and we had a great relationship, that would later, become like family. I handed him the DVD of almost everything we experienced and told him the camera was loaned to me by my dear friend Dr. Rubin. He wished us well and left. What a grand gesture of him, I thought, to not only call but be there in person to share in our departure, which he knew was a glorious and happy occasion for PaviElle and our family.

Some say lawyers are cold and only in it for the money, but Ron Rosen proved that to be false. He showed us so much love, care and gave me thoughtful advice like a father would. His son Evon who joined the legal team later on has become like a brother and someone who truly cares about my daughter.

They say that Murphy's Law will always get you, but in my case even the simple delivery of the items necessary for PaviElle's home care was botched. Some items were delivered and some, like feeding pump with bags were delivered but with no cord or formula, and there was no commode nor bath chair. Hence, I had to be on the telephone nonstop until everything was sorted out. We were going home the next day, but more challenges were definitely ahead, from Medicaid, to formula, wheel chair, nurse and home health aide. As I look back I wonder how my body and mind survived. It could only have been God giving me inner strength.

Chapter 8

e left Jackson Memorial Hospital's Rehabilitation Unit on the 29th of August 2007 and it suddenly dawned on me that it was on May 29th, three months past that I took my child to the emergency room of a Palm Beach Hospital and she was admitted. With tears in my eyes I looked around the very small room and half bathroom to make sure we were leaving nothing behind. We then walked down the hallway, hearing screams of children left behind, to the gorgeous outdoors filled with sunshine. We were extremely happy to be finally going home. Lloyd loaded the car while I kept hugging and kissing a smiling PaviElle who was without doubt the happiest person in the world. We captured the moment on video but it has been etched in my mind, even now as I write it, to share with you. The nurses and some staff members came to the car to bid us farewell and emotions were high as they all cried with joy and wished us good luck. They asked us to come back to visit when she returned for follow up visits to see Dr. Podda.

When we drove away PaviElle cheered and it filled my heart. The journey quickly went by and she called out all the landmarks she remembered. Those places we thought were significant we pointed out to her. It was incredible. At that moment I thought little about good student with great grades and doing all the things, like golf and tennis, that she loved and did so well before she was stricken.

We stopped at a pharmacy to drop off the numerous prescriptions but found out that some were not covered by Medicaid and had to be omitted. When we eventually turned into the drive way of our house, PaviElle's face was a picture of profound joy and happiness. She had made the long journey without a bathroom accident, and proudly she proclaimed that to us. When we got inside she directed her dad to place her in her favorite chair, the one at the sliding door then she asked to be switched to another chair, and declared emphatically, "God is going to make me walk again."

Later she asked to go into her bed. As she looked at her pictures on the wall she said, "I'm so cute I'm going to be good again. I'm going to be well." I had taken lots of her photo albums to the hospital and kept reminding her of how she looked before with long hair, since she was now bald. We had also shown her pictures of her room, the house; friends and relatives so she would not forget, the things and people she loved. Without warning, she burst out in a deep, heart wrenching sob, then asked me, "Why in the world did this happen to me, why did I get so sick?"

Instantly, I felt depressed but, tried my best to explain to her that anyone can get sick and that she definitely would be well again. I asked Lloyd to explain the same thing to her, and with both our explanation she stopped crying. She then talked a lot more and her speech became clearer as evening turned to night, and during the said she wanted to use the toilet for a bowel movement but we were too slow in getting her out of bed to the toilet so she started too soon, but we allowed her to finish on the toilet. We cleaned her, brought her back to bed and congratulated her several times for using the toilet successfully. She asked her dad not to go to work and then fell asleep again. However, Lloyd had to leave for work, which made her feel lonely and sad when she awoke. Later that day, a nurse named Jim visited from an agency (Home Is Where The Heart Is). He gave her all the medications, cleaned the G Tube and changed the dressing on her toes. While she slept we signed all the tons of forms that felt like being admitted to the hospital again.

The day went well, then Jim was off on his revved-up motor cycle. PaviElle did not seem to like him much so I was happy when I received a call from a lady named Connie who was apparently the person the hospital had sent PaviElle's file. We were to get another nurse from another agency that Connie provided. This exercise would prove to be so stressful and frustrating to the point where I just wanted to say forget it. I was informed that the services of the nurse would only last for a few weeks, and a home-health aide would be provided for thirty days. How would I manage, I worried, when these services ended? However, the good Lord God intervened again and sent us a wonderful woman, named Ms. Suzanne. She was tall, big framed and looked strong, with a beautiful smile and great personality. She was just the person we needed. PaviElle was resistant to her at first, but after she gave her a second bath, she began to like her. The first bath she got was frightening for her, because she was afraid of the water and the shower. When Lloyd and I had tried to give her a shower

Jackson PICU, and who always called to see how we were managing. The reason for her visit was to deliver all the forms necessary for homebound school. I was required to fill them out and fax them to Suzie at Jackson Memorial Rehab for Dr. Restrepo the rehab doctor to sign and return.

When Ms. Parrado saw PaviElle her sadness was visible but she again related her story of when she was married and suffered a brain injury. She said, "Remember, I was much older and married, so if I can recover PaviElle will also."

With those encouraging words of advice, I thanked her and she left. It was extremely difficult for me when someone who knew PaviElle before her illness visited because you could see the shock on their faces realizing that she weighed only 76 pounds, her head completely bald and her eyes looked wild and piercing. She was not the beautiful, unusually long hair girl, with the perfect weight that they knew and admired.

On our second day home, PaviElle was again crying, saying she was hungry, and the twitching she had in the hospital returned. The nurse did not come that day so I had to deal with the situation on my own, give all the medications, and then change the dressing on her toes. I quickly became an expert therapist, nurse and teacher, because I realized there would be days like this when no one would show up. To pass the time each day I gathered up all her FCAT tests. I had her try to do the comprehension first and to my surprise she did great reading the stories and able to relate to me what she read.

hard every day on every subject, and the words she struggled to pronounce, especially those words with the D sound, until the home-school teacher came.

It was now time to tackle the outpatient therapy. I called Health South and spoke to Cathy the physical therapist. I wanted to get information about their equipment for walking and swallowing. However, the short conversation proved futile. When I called back to set up the therapy appointments I was informed that Medicaid was not accepted and CMS who would pay was voluntarily assigned by the hospital, therefore it was all a no go. I was livid and in a state of disbelief. I called Donna the administrator, and Suzie the nurse practitioner in charge of rehab, at Jacksons and then Ruth the nurse. Nothing happened and no one knew why. I was given a number by Bridgette, the social worker from the sixth floor at Jackson Memorial, but no one answered and Bridgette was now on vacation. "What a trying day!" I yelled, cried and screamed out to God.

In the midst of all this chaos and confusion, PaviElle asked me why her foot looked so black and dirty and about the huge scar on her thigh. I had to stop and explain again what happened to her at the hospital in Palm Beach. She seemed to understand but I wasn't too

I continued to work with her as best as I could. She was sitting up with pillows but kept falling over and drooling from her mouth, and was still not swallowing and continued to cry for hunger. The doctors at the hospital had told me that she would not remember the

the names of the students she recognized. The banner was arranged by Mr. Bender in collaboration with Dr. Rubin. This was a wonderful break for us to enjoy. During the visit I realized while trying to move her from the chair to the wheelchair that it had no seatbelt so she kept sliding out. The wheelchair was extremely heavy and unmanageable for me, so I called the company and spoke with Rolando who said she could do nothing.

The other complaint was that the feed formula they sent had expired, and I could not believe that the dietitian at Jackson recommended a formula with corn to replace one with corn. I came to the conclusion that they figured if you are a Medicaid patient you must be stupid and don't read labels.

I called Marie from United Health Care and told her of my frustrations, road blocks and disappointments. She empathized with me and promised to contact a therapy company near my house that would possibly take PaviElle for all three disciplines of therapy. I waited anxiously for her call and she came through with Advance Pediatrics, a therapy company some twenty minutes from my house. I thanked her repeatedly and immediately called the center. I spoke to Linda who said she needed to discuss the case with her director and promised to call me back the next day.

When Lloyd got home, we decided to take PaviElle to the Wellington Mall. When we got to the mall and put her in the wheelchair, she was happy but seemed afraid of the people walking around. She also kept sliding out of the chair since it had no belt. I noticed she had

When we returned home I called the company about the wheelchair again and was told if a patient only had Medicaid, this was the chair Medicaid paid for, so everyone with Medicaid got the same chair. I thought of the saying I heard from childhood - "Poverty is a crime."

Daphne the new nurse that was assigned called very late to say she would see us the next day. She also said they told her that I knew everything PaviElle needed so I would show her what to do. Interesting I thought before I struggled to fall asleep.

That night PaviElle got totally soaked with the formula as the feed went flying everywhere in the room including the ceiling. I had to clean her up again. While I was doing this she told me, "I can sleep in my own bed," and also said she remembered the home and cell numbers. I granted her command and went to my own bed, but sleep was far off, so I decided to watch TV.

As I watched CNN there was a story about New Orleans. It was reported that during Hurricane Katrina nurses used Morphine and Versed to euthanize patients. I immediately called and left a message for our attorney, Ron Rosen, regarding the report I was watching. He returned my call the next morning and promised to order a transcript of the report.

The new nurse came late at 11:00 a.m. after I already gave PaviElle all her medications that were due at 10:00 a.m. Suzanne the home health aide had arrived on time at 10:00 a.m. and gave her a good shower. It was our first holiday weekend spent at home, so we had sweet girl as she said with a smirk on her face "She's so skinny."

The young woman had to be almost forced to go to my daughter's room to say hello. I felt so hurt by that incident and worried deeply about the problems she would face at school when she was well enough to return. PaviElle asked to sleep with us in our bed and we allowed her to. However, I noticed that she was running a temperature, which I assumed was due to the fact that she had been exposed to so many people during the day. I gave her Tylenol and the fever went away. As the saying goes, "There is no rest for the weary," as next day I resumed the numerous phone calls to try and solve the issue with CMS paying for the therapies. I finally was able to speak with Bridgette the social worker from Jackson, but she could give me no answers. I tried Mary Anne from CMS again, but was still unable to reach her. I was once more becoming really frustrated calling so many people with hardly any result.

I was convinced that October would be the month that out-patient therapy would begin, so I called and spoke to Sharon the director at Advanced Pediatrics to tell her my daughter's tragic story and discovered she had a niece who had suffered a similar fate of a negligent doctor and a hospital error at birth. She tried very hard to give me comfort and hope on the phone and I was confident she would do her utmost best to give PaviElle a slot at the center, even though, she mentioned they were full to capacity. It is so wonderful when God steps in and make what seems impossible, possible, when you believe and trust Him. The good news came when Linda from Advance Pediatrics called in the same afternoon to say I could bring diapers, chucks or wipes, which were some of the items absolutely necessary for PaviElle's home care. I was also told that I had to pick a plan with CMS, but I had no idea what plan to pick. In my confusion I again called Marie from United Health Care for advice on picking a plan with CMS. I was astonished that the system is filled with so many twists and turns that one is forced to navigate, while one is in the midst of such tragedies and devastations like a serious illness of a loved one.

Over and over I wondered if anyone really cared. But I remained relentless, refusing to crumble under the weight of the system. I tried doing some research to find a patient advocate but only reached a dead end. The best news of that day was that PaviElle sat up by herself for half an hour, then one hour. She did exercises with and without weights and she stood up twice. This made my day super. Lloyd came home and saw her sitting up and kept thanking the Lord.

When we arrived at Advance Pediatrics the next day I thought therapy would begin but again I had to swing into action, because the approved, signed forms that were sent to Jackson Rehab for Dr. Restrepo's signature had not been re-faxed to the center. I broke down so bad that they had to take me into a private room to comfort me until I stopped bawling. I then gathered myself and got on the telephone calling several times until I got Suzie at Jackson. She kept trying to get me off the telephone and said she would fax the forms but I insisted that I would not hang up until I saw the forms coming through the fax machine.

would be given three sessions per week of each therapy - physical, occupational and speech.

Moving on to the next phase would bring the same level of frustration and disappointment. I was told to call Palms West Hospital because they had a speech therapist named Yvette who was excellent for the video swallow procedure. This would be the first step in making sure it was safe for PaviElle to swallow and subsequently start eating again. I kept calling and calling, leaving several messages with no response. I decided to call the director, Bob, whose name I had to try very hard to get. He invited me to tour the facility for which he gave rave reviews, and so I did. I struggled to put PaviElle and the wheel chair in the car by myself and we went to visit Palms West. The tour was educational and we met all the therapists including the elusive Yvette that I had tried so hard to reach, and she was impressive and seemed very knowledgeable about her work. All this was great until I received a telephone call from the registration department stating that Palms West no longer accepted United Health Care insurance. I was pissed.

As soon as we got back home, Linda from Advance Pediatrics was calling to fax me more forms to fill out. My life had become a sea of paper work that should be shunned by anyone even slightly concerned about the environment.

Concerned about the video swallow procedure I then called JFK Hospital in Palm Beach County but learned they only did therapy for eighteen year olds and up. Ms. Ferquson called from Medicaid at last her the enrollment form because she was out of office at a meeting. I had called her so many times and left so many messages she was forced to return my call. I called to thank her, after Ms. Ferguson called me from Medicaid. I also called and left several messages after Paula told me she would be the person receiving the form and granting the approval.

A synopsis of PaviElle's tragic story was left on everyone's voice mail until I got results. I was relentless in my efforts to get the help my only child needed to help with her recovery. Soon the short tenure of the nurse that was assigned to PaviElle ended, and Suzanne the aide was also scheduled to leave soon, as her thirty days was fast approaching. I tried desperately to get an extension of the time for Suzanne because she had become such a great help with PaviElle's

I called Dr. Podda and Suzie at Jackson until I began to think they were tired of hearing my voice. They politely tried to convince me otherwise and did what they could to help. Talking to Suzie one day after trying to jump over so many hurdles, running into road blocks and having so many disappointments, I told her I felt like, "Killing myself" because I was overwhelmed with grief. I sat in my room and sobbed with her on the telephone feeling so overwhelmed and defeated. She begged me to stay on the phone until she could talk me out of the low that I was experiencing. She kept reminding me that if I was not such a caring and loving mother PaviElle would not have lived. She begged me not to give up hope and to rid my mind of such severe thoughts. I stayed on the telephone so long with Suzie bawl and nights when my pillow was so wet with tears, it had to be turned over. But I steadfastly asked God to give me strength to cope and overcome all the turbulence and destruction my life was going through at the moment. This was the first and only time from the day the tragedy happened that suicide had entered my mind. Thank the Lord it never occurred again.

PaviElle would continue to have good days in therapy and her ability to swallow slowly got better, as well as the strength of her tongue. My friends, Dr. Rubin, Joan and Judy visited often, but I did not allow myself to share with them the hard times I was having because I never wanted pity.

A few days after returning home, Lloyd and I ventured out on our second visit with PaviElle to the mall. We went to Palm Beach Lakes for a visit to the Sears's store there, a place we hoped she would remember, and she did.

With regard to the video swallow I told myself it was God's will to delay the procedure. PaviElle was talking more in therapy at the center. She told Suzanne, the aide, when she tried to tell her to do something, "Only my mommy and daddy must tell me what to do." We were all shocked.

Our next road trip to Whole Foods at Gardens Mall was also successful and good for restoring her memory. The therapy was going great and physical therapy with Janet was being done at home some days so she could help PaviElle to get in and out of bed. This took a while

On her first day, the 17th, she was absolutely impressive. She was the one that would make her eat again. We began to make progress with Malissa but PaviElle started to become afraid of swallowing food. Malissa persevered, until she became her favorite therapist, knocking Janet into second place. That was also the day when she marched, raised her toes, shook her hands up and down, wrote her name with a marker, then drew circles, lines down and across. The next day we would have great news to share with Dr. Podda, as we journeyed back to Jackson for her first follow up visit. He was extremely happy to see the progress she had made since leaving the hospital. He kept telling Lloyd how great a mother I was, and called Dr. Fernandez and Jennifer to see PaviElle. They were very surprised to see her improvements and were in tears. We visited the nurses on the sixth floor who also cried and looked on with disbelief.

The visit to PICU was also dramatic as Dr. Narez saw us at the door and came running out. When he saw PaviElle he hugged her and with tears in his eyes he said to my mom, who had accompanied us, "Your daughter is a wonderful mom and is responsible for PaviElle's recovery." I told him he had also played a part along with the other doctors and with God's help. I knew my mom felt a great sense of pride and joy.

The 21st of September would also lead to another great journey that would accelerate PaviElle's recovery. Ms. Bins from the Palm Beach School Board Homebound School Department called to set a meeting at my house for 8:30 a.m. that morning. I agreed but felt apprehensive because I knew I would be alone with PaviElle that named Scottish Rights Children Hospital with a great program, but it was in Atlanta. She related several incidences of the program's success, where children who had suffered brain injuries from Palm Beach School District had gone to the facility and returned with nothing short of a miraculous success. She gave me the name of a woman named Mimi Gold at the facility, and a telephone number for her. I thanked her and they left.

As soon as I closed the door I started dialing the number. I left numerous messages but had no response. I kept calling and after several weeks I eventually got Mimi on the telephone. She apologized profusely and explained that she was on vacation and had just finished listening to my desperate messages. She explained the procedure to get into the general program but was not sure which specific program would be suitable for PaviElle. She was only the teacher she said. She gave me another number to get more detailed information and immediately I began calling again. Meanwhile, Dr. Podda called with the results of the various blood tests and X Ray done at the follow up visit at Jackson and reported that all was well. We would see him in another few months.

I kept calling Atlanta every day, several times per day. When I did get to speak to someone I discovered the procedure to get PaviElle admitted for therapy wasn't a simple task. I had to get letters of recommendation from the rehab doctors at Jackson, then, her pediatrician, Dr. Chan, who would have to write a letter giving authorization and approval so that Medicaid would pay for intense therapy in another state. I managed to make all the requests and was needed from the therapists at Advance Pediatric System.

It took another long period of time to get all the therapists to meet and then each write progress reports along with a single letter with all their signatures. This I considered a major undertaking and a drawn out task, but one I was determined to complete.

After getting all the letters I realized that the most crucial one from Dr. Chan the Pediatrician, needed to allow for payment from Medicaid was not there. I called the lady at his office who was taking care of the letter and she told me Dr. Chan could not write the letter because it would not help. I was devastated. I got on the computer immediately and started to do some research and found out that we literally had to move to the State of Georgia, although PaviElle was declared disabled and brain damaged in order for Medicaid to pay for her therapy at the hospital in Atlanta. Without hesitation, I knew we had no choice but to move the family to Atlanta. Luckily my mom lives there so I could move in with her. A few more hurdles would have to be jumped before we moved. Malissa, the speech pathologist had to give the green light for the video swallow, and the G Tube had to be removed surgically at Jackson, using Propofol to put PaviElle to sleep. All these procedures were frightening, because anything could potentially go very wrong including the closure of the wound once the G Tube was removed. I was told that if the hole did not close in three days we would have to return to the hospital for follow up. Miraculously the hole was closed the next morning and I called Charlene immediately to tell her the miraculous news. She was so elated and happy for me.

her good advice and counsel. PaviElle had become so attached to Janet that one day when she had to go out of town and asked Renee to do the PT session, she gave Renee a hard time. She screamed and cried the entire session and on our way home she was sad but kept repeating my entire name, over and over. That night the same thing continued. She apologized to me for her behavior and I hugged her, telling her it was okay to cry and express her feelings. The occupational therapist made a splint for her left hand to keep it open but she refused to wear it at nights. She managed to take it off every night and I was beginning to feel frustrated and mad as I watched her struggle with the simple things she use to do without even thinking about it.

Dr. Rubin became my savior when she came to visit and I broke down and wept as she hugged me. She tried her best to provide words of comfort and encouragement. As usual, she would bring something to challenge PaviElle's brain, read stories with her and gave me a break.

On October 1, 2007 CMS Medi Pass clicked in, although I wasn't sure what difference it would make in the scheme of things. However, I found out quickly when Malissa asked me to get a prescription from the doctor for a spirometer and United Health Care refused to pay for it. I called Paula at CMS and she approved the payment so we could get the device. To this day PaviElle continues to use it in speech therapy. The next day, PaviElle stood up on her own for the first time and did not even realize it. Malissa worked hard to get her to eat several things including mashed potatoes, jelly, brown sugar an evaluation. This would take a much longer time to happen than I anticipated, but we continued to plan on moving.

Her recovery was actually in high gear and we visited Dr. Chan for the first general check up since PaviElle was stricken. He was blown away when he came into the exam room and saw that she PaviElle was so skinny and sitting in a wheel chair. He tried to hold his emotions together and asked Lloyd to lift her unto the table. He examined her and gave us encouragement about the possibility of recovery from brain injuries. He referred us to Dr. Friedman an ophthalmologist and Dr. Lue a pediatric neurologist.

Another block would arise when PaviElle wanted to use the computer. She was doing so well with everything else and I decided to allow her to sit at the computer. In retrospect I think it was a mistake. After a few minutes she began to scream and look afraid and then her eyes seemed out of focus. I called Dr. Chan but it was after 5:00 p.m. I explained to the nurse what was happening and that I suspected PaviElle was having a seizure. She advised me to take her to the emergency room. However, she had fallen asleep while I was on the telephone. When she woke up she asked to use the bathroom but as I was trying to sit her up to stand up and then go to the bathroom she had a seizure. I called 911 immediately, but the paramedics took like what seemed like an eternity to arrive, even though they were about twenty-five minutes away. The seizure stopped long before the Fire Rescue truck arrived with the sound of the siren and a loud knock on the door that made me realize they had arrived. It was such a nerve racking experience, I think I lost all my nerves for a moment.

some attention and medication. The nurse said the usual "I'm sorry" a phrase I have grown to hate. Then came the nurse practitioner, then the doctor who entered with his pompous persona and no apology. He gave her Adavant and then Phenobaub that knocked her out. I became nervous thinking of the Versed that also had the same effect at the other hospital that started all this tragedy.

While talking to the nurse, Tracy, and telling her what happened to her at the other Palm Beach hospital, her comment was, "We are getting a lot of people coming here, telling us such bad things about that hospital. Why would they give your daughter Versed when she was having trouble breathing? Both Versed and Adavant are drugs that will put you into Cardiac Arrest." As she said this she looked at me with sadness in her eyes.

Eventually, PaviElle was admitted and taken to a room for the night. All the nurses wanted to hear our story and they did their best to care for her and made us comfortable. The next morning PaviElle had an EEG but Dr. Lue the Neurologist said she did not need to have an MRI since she had one in June at Jackson Memorial. He requested the medical records. All this was done by telephone, but he came to see us later in the afternoon and prescribed 2.5ml of Triliptol and explained what to do if she had another seizure. During our conversation his cell phone rang and I noticed he looked disturbed and was getting annoyed. I asked him if something was wrong, and he said, "I cannot believe this, they made me see the wrong baby at the hospital."

said she was hungry on our way home so I knew she was feeling

Malissa came the next day, but PaviElle was not herself. She seemed limp and somewhat weak, so we tried to make her eat. Malissa saw the depressed state I was in, and told me not to worry, assuring me PaviElle would be okay soon. I tried very hard to make her relax and she fell asleep, waking up more energetic and asked to play Monopoly her favorite board game.

We played for a very long time as she didn't want to stop. In the midst of my exhaustion she fell asleep and the phone rang. To my relief it was Prophetess Peart. I thanked God she called at a time when I really needed to hear her voice. She always called at the perfect and on-time moment, when I am about to enter the deep dark and dreary hole of depression, trying to soothe myself with a huge pity-party.

I decided to move to another gear to test PaviElle's memory by taking her to all familiar places and see if she remembered them. For example, she requested Dunkin Donuts, so on the way there I drove on the street where my friend Judy's house was located and asked who lived there, and she quickly replied without hesitation, "Auntie Judy." She of course wanted to visit. We got the donuts and as we entered the complex I asked who lives in another house we were approaching she said "Auntie Barbara." This was a happy moment, and the visit to Judy's was great for her. She did all the things she would normally do at Judy's house, looked in the pantry, used the computer and did not want to leave. When we got home she did she could not walk; she inspected my clothes, sat and searched a basket she loved, and then looked in the pantry. I was very busy giving her the tour of the house in her wheel chair and sometimes holding her to try walking. Later she wanted to be taken back to the pantry, where she picked out a pack of her Ramen noodles and asked me to prepare it for her. I did, but she only ate a tiny amount. Next she asked to be taken to the freezer to get ice cream and she had some. With all this activity she kept me on my toes.

Prophetess and her prayer team were coming for their first home visit so I decided to surprise them. When they rang the bell I was holding PaviElle so she could stand at the island in the kitchen to have her ice cream. I crazily placed her hand so she could hold on to the counter and ran to the door. I said to my visitors, "Come, come, quickly. You must see this."

They rushed in and saw PaviElle standing at the island and trying to feed herself, for the first time since she had taken sick, with the ice cream. They were ecstatic, euphoric, happy, celebrating and thanking God all at the same time. This was a glorious moment of hope and complete joy in her recovery process. We had a wonderful Holy Spirit-filled prayer meeting which my husband missed (the reason would be revealed to me later in a phone call from a stranger). They blessed the entire house and anointed me with oil. I gave an offering to the church, something I always chose to do because it was the right thing. This was not a payment, but for me showing appreciation for them to take time out of their busy schedules to visit my home and pray for my daughter and family.

was so good at before the brain injury. I continued to vigorously pursue the move to Atlanta with a great sense of urgency so I decided to do more research about the brain. I recalled when I pursued my course in interior design that my professor taught about the effects of color on the brain and learning. I called the professor and asked if she would loan me the text book that she lectured from on the subject, and she was very happy to do so.

When I got the book and read it every moment I had to spare, my answer was revealed. The colors clearly showed which color affected learning on each section of the brain. I called my husband and asked that we all go to Lowes or Home Depot to purchase purple and blue no VOC (volatile organic compounds) paint, to paint PaviElle's new room. He was skeptical and resistant because he dislikes painting. We got the paint and switched PaviElle to the bigger room and painted non-stop until the job was complete. I had to explain to Lloyd the method to my madness and what the different colors meant to the

For me it was very simple. Purple is for stimulating intuition, imagination and creativity and blue is relaxing, calming, lower blood pressure, regulates sleep and is also linked to the throat and thyroid. Once the painting was complete and all the large furniture pieces transferred to the larger room, I used my interior design skills to decorate the room, adding other colors like green and splashes of red and black.

We returned her to the repainted and newly designed room and the results were obvious the next morning. 'This is awesome," I thought,

Deadly Negligence 111

She began eating more of the things she liked in the past in small portions. Because of her low weight, just 76 pounds, we provided her with anything she asked to eat. I also placed her on a juice and nourishing soup regimen. No processed foods were allowed, everything was made from scratch because I was told her body needed to be cleansed of the chemo and would heal faster and better. I was on full throttle.

All of this must have been very effective because shortly after this my neighbor Roberta came to visit. She decided to sit with PaviElle and go through all our photo albums to see who she recognized.

In the midst of that October 16, 2007 evening PaviElle STOOD UP and WALKED to her room. We were jubilant and I kept screaming, 'Thank you Jesus, Thank you Jesus," dancing and shouting for joy.

Roberta quickly got up and followed her to her room in a state of shock to make sure she was safe and did not fall but that was definitely not necessary. She began going through her closet, searching through her baskets, looking at her jewelry and asking for her jewelry box that I had hidden while she was hospitalized. I made the decision not to call Lloyd and share the new miracle, but waited for him to come home and experience his own surprise and jubilation.

As he entered the den I called PaviElle to come to me. He looked puzzled and confused, obviously wondering why I was calling her and she could not walk and why was she in her room by herself. As she walked into the den, he dropped the contents in his hand, of God's miracles in PaviElle's life. I kept saying, "I told you all, that God is still in the miracle working business and will come through for her. She will be totally healed in the name of Jesus," recalling the words of the sign I posted over her bed when she was in the hospital. I thought of all the doubters we had to deal with in the hospital and even my mom who was hopeful but skeptical.

I had refused to listen to any negative words about her total recovery. I chose to only believe in God's might, even on those dark days and nights when I was alone with my thoughts and shedding my river of

The next morning at 5:15 a.m. PaviElle managed to navigate her way in the dark to our bedroom. I was lying in my bed praying, but could hear her through the baby monitor we had placed on her night table getting out of her bed. She had gotten out of bed, put her slippers on, the one we bought at TJ Maxx, and walked straight to our room. She stood on my side of the bed and announced, "Mommy and Daddy I'm here, look at me."

I jumped out of bed and hugged her tight and kissed her cheeks. Lloyd who can normally sleep through a fire and a storm jumped up and was again in total disbelief. I said aloud to the Lord, "This is a great day you have made, we will rejoice and be glad in it." She made more progress when she wrote her name clearly, then drank water from a bottle for the first time since she began to recover.

My spirit was high so I decided to call Social Security about a letter

She further explained that Jackson Memorial should have sent Social Security Administration a Release Letter to say PaviElle had been discharged and therefore put in motion an increase in the amount we should have been receiving for being at home. She told me not to worry because the money would be paid retroactively and my daughter was entitled to it because of her disability and brain injury status. I was really surprised because I was totally unaware of this, as it wasn't in my realm of thought or possibility. Who knew that my only child would have suffered in this way? I then took the opportunity to tell her about the intense therapy she needed and available in Atlanta.

Again she gave me great information about the rights of my daughter based on her disability status and the fact that Medicaid would pay for the therapy. I took her advice and speeded up my efforts for the move to Atlanta. I also called Jackson and spoke with Eddie. He had no idea about the Release Letter, so I told him to call the Social Security office at Jackson and they would tell him about the letter and exactly what to write. He accepted my suggestion, got the letter and faxed it off to me the next day. I was grateful for the financial intervention through Social Security because we desperately needed money to buy all the medical supplies and medications that PaviElle needed to help speed up her recovery. Lloyd's small electrical business that was doing so well while I was doing marketing for the company, had fallen flat on its face and our funds were extremely low. Thankfully, we had my mom and a kind hearted family friend who sent us money to help buy petrol for our long daily journeys, taken mostly by Lloyd, since I lived at the hospital. PaviElle kept reaching milestones like she was

She even tried to make her bed again and called me to inspect it. It was obviously not perfect but I celebrated her effort. Her big personal celebration came when she started to wear panties again. She was so elated and filled with pride. I knew what she experienced was great embarrassment and shame especially when we had visitors or her dad had to change her diaper. She was now going to the bathroom on her own, although she was still having difficulty pulling her panties down and up. She was also trying very hard to dress herself and using the knife and fork to eat, and improving her writing, She told the occupational therapist, Nicole, that she had spelt her first name incorrectly, with a lower case e instead of an upper case E. That was also something she had told my friend Joan one Christmas when she was five years old, when she took PaviElle to buy her a bracelet and wrote her name with a small e instead of an upper case E. Joan was shocked at her persistence then about the correct spelling of her name. Her nightlight was her next joy when she plugged it in and started singing Spanish songs she knew.

At last, the long awaited call came from Atlanta to have an appointment for PaviElle to see the physiatrist Dr. Johnson and be evaluated to determine if she was a good candidate for the intense therapy rehab. Words cannot explain my feelings as I heard the voice of the lady on the telephone. I could not contain my joy so I exploded with praise and thanksgiving.

I took PaviElle to see the neurologist Dr. Lue, and he discontinued all medications and said she looked great and was progressing well. She was no longer wetting her panties at nights, and was now setting

Deadly Negligence 115

her own after use. This was good as it showed she was gaining back her strength. I began to take her out visiting and shopping much more often which helped her memory and recovery.

Therapy was also accelerated because the school board was testing her to determine her eligibility for speech therapy, paid for and provided through the school system for disabled students. The test administered by Mary took so long that PaviElle looked totally exhausted. After an hour and-a-half I was forced to stop the test. It seemed so ridiculous because by looking at PaviElle and noticing that when Mary tried talking to her she could barely communicate, it should have been obvious that she needed the speech therapy provided by the school district. When I questioned Mary she explained that this was her first case, and even though it was obvious that PaviElle was disabled and needed the therapy, it had to be done.

That day I clearly understood that in government people are not able to use judgment. The completion of the test was rescheduled for the next morning, and she qualified for the speech therapy. Dr. Lue decided to stop all medications after she did an EEG in his office. She was also progressing with homebound school especially with Math. That day was good news from all sides, but the next day would be fantastic.

Chapter 9

n November 7, 2007 we were moving to Atlanta. This was not a move that we really wanted to make but had to if PaviElle was going to get the intense therapy that everyone recommended. I was told, that with the speed of her recovery she needed to go to a facility that offered that type of treatment in order for her to continue moving forward. They were all right.

We had to drive the ten hour journey, because PaviElle was very scared of flying. When we arrived she remembered her grandmother's house and the city in general. She also recognized the inside of the house but was terrified of the stairs. I was surprised about her fear of the staircase because that was a feature she really loved and enjoyed in the past. Her strength improved and she was able to open and close the car door. She also started to point out cars on the road that looked like her grandmother's.

Lloyd and I went downtown Atlanta to the Social Security office, following the instructions given to us from the lady I spoke with on the telephone back in Florida. God provided us with an excellent counselor, who was very thorough and patient. She gave us the letter

The following day would be a major one. We finally met Sharon, Dr. Johnson's nurse who I had been communicating with for weeks. The interview was extremely emotional for me because I had to relate the tragic story from the beginning to Sharon and then repeat it for Dr. Johnson. When he entered the room, I felt a great feeling of relief and calm, even before he started the evaluation. As I told him the details of the tragedy, my tears came tumbling down and PaviElle and Lloyd tried to console me. When he completed the evaluation he looked us straight in the eyes and said "She is the perfect candidate for our program."

In unison, we said "Thank you God."

Nurse Sharon then took us for a tour of both the in-patient and out-patient facilities. They were both impressive. We were then in the next phase of paperwork and all the things we needed before being given a start date.

Janet, PaviElle's physical therapist from Florida, called to find out if she had gotten accepted into the program. We gave her the good news and she was ecstatic. The evening provided another element of joy, when PaviElle's friend Simone called, and later she took her first shower with me since she had been so ill. God is truly great. It was just a succession of miracles.

Being in Atlanta was therapeutic for PaviElle because she loved Georgia. My friend Laverne and her children James and Katelan came to visit and the most amazing thing happened. The stairs that clear to me; my sweet girl was coming back.

When we realized that it would take a few weeks before starting the program at Children's Health Care of Atlanta we decided to go back to Florida to move more things. My mother came with us to assist with the little she can do, because she is also disabled. We left Atlanta for the long journey but Lloyd got a ticket in a construction area. I was upset but we took it in stride and enjoyed the trip. PaviElle was an absolute trooper both going to Atlanta and back to Florida. I had worried unnecessarily, about her needing to use the bathroom and getting exhausted from the long travel time. When we returned it was necessary to see the school psychologist for testing. The results showed that her IQ was average even with the brain injury. This was great news so we needed to focus on perceptive thinking and

I began to focus on teaching her Spanish and French. I used video tapes, audio, picture books, television and radio to infiltrate her mind and test the research that learning a foreign language is good for the brain's recovery. The results were evident. It was obvious her brain was being challenged and her memory was improving. The school board also required her to do a hearing and vision test even though we were moving to Atlanta. The therapist apologized for doing the test because it was her first time doing it.

PaviElle was now looking better, her lips looked normal, and Dr. Podda was again extremely surprised by her continued recovery, especially that she was walking on her own. He kept asking me what

Deadly Negligence

call with the date when she would start the program in Atlanta, and possibly having to cut off the tip of her toe, that was so black and severely scarred.

Roberta my neighbor, and her granddaughters, were going to the new library in Wellington and invited PaviElle to go along with them. I decided to go and she had a fantastic time.

With all this going on, I began to notice a change in my husband's attitude, raising his voice, being impatient and late coming home. He started saying crazy things like, "You are both treating me like an alien," and, "You only think about yourself."

I couldn't believe my ears. Another incident occurred at the dining table when PaviElle declared she would be on the Food Network one day. I was surprised by Lloyd's negative reaction, but used the opportunity to ask him why he was so mean and tired when he came home. In a very firm tone he said "I am not."

I reminded him about what he said earlier and he said he did not remember. I then tried to get PaviElle to confirm what I was saying, but instead she said, "Mom, I'm trying to eat here, and I would like to eat my food in peace."

I then decided that her total recovery was so much bigger, more important and urgent than to be distracted by Lloyd's strange behavior and seeming infidelity. PaviElle needed my undivided attention and focus, to endure the extremely long and emotional the music, she responded in a very firm tone, "I am not exactly deaf Mom." Then I would ask about places we lived like Rochdale Village in Queens, New York and she asked "Why wouldn't I remember?"

Chapter 10

On November 21, 2007 we were on our way back to Atlanta, hoping to get the most anticipated phone call from Children's Health Care of Atlanta. I tried my best to not display any visible anxiety about the wait but inside all I could think about was the phone ringing and it would be someone with a friendly voice giving me a date.

We went to a family friend, Ms. Smith, to celebrate my favorite holiday, Thanksgiving. She was so happy to see PaviElle's recovery in person that she said seeing her made her day. The day became even better when PaviElle recognized everyone at the dinner and remembered the jokes and family stories revived by Ms. Smith pertaining to her brother who had died previously. We all had a great time.

The next day, Black Friday, we decided to take her out to get shoes which was somewhat overwhelming at first but eventually, we managed to get what she needed. This adventure also provided a much needed spark to her memory, as the store was a place she really loved, prior to the tragedy. I was happy, but felt sad all the time and cried myself to sleep every night, thinking about all she had lost and her daily constant struggle.

with basic things like going to the bathroom. Laverne assured me that she would be fine and reminded me that she was a nurse. I thanked her and began to cry, with tears of gratitude.

As I relate this event my tears still flow and my heart aches. Mr. Bender also called and offered to continue reading to PaviElle by telephone since we were now living in Atlanta. He talked to her and then did what he always does, prayed. She began to crave foods she had loved in the past and rummaged through all her old belongings. We were both blue because Lloyd had to return to Florida for work and to tie up other commitments.

I lost my patience and took matters in my own hands and called CHA to get a date for starting the intense rehab program. I left several messages, no one called me back that day but my action would produce results. The following morning, I received the very important call that would prove to be all that it was supposed to be. I called everyone and gave them the great news. Melissa, the speech therapist who played such a significant role in making PaviElle eat again, expressed her disappointment for not being part of her continued recovery. PaviElle had that effect on everyone involved in her recovery, they all wanted to be involved in her future, because her story was so tragic and devastating.

Dr. Rubin volunteered to teach her Spanish on the phone to keep her mind active because our moving stopped the math and science lessons she taught her on all the wonderful visits to her house. PaviElle began to do so well, it gave my mom courage to take her to early and waited for a while. Things seemed a bit disorganized, we had to change location but was taken to the gymnasium where Lisa the occupational therapist came to see PaviElle.

Next, it was time for Kim the physical therapist and Loretta, the nurse who became a great source of help, caring and encouraging. Loretta was the person I could call anytime to apprehend my fears and dispel my doubts.

She took extra special care of my daughter, treated her as if she was her own child. At the end of the program she gave PaviElle a gold bracelet that is worn and treasured with appreciation. Jason, the speech pathologist seemed good at his job, but PaviElle never had a male therapist, and we wondered if he would be as effective, smart and thorough as Malissa.

Dr. Rubin called from Florida to hear how the first day went at the center. I had good news because PaviElle appeared to be walking better after the first day. I cried a lot on this day, some for joy and some for sorrow. I had to give God the Glory, when she told me the day was enjoyable and she preferred it to Florida. She was visibly exhausted but happy.

The second day I was still blue and got to meet the teacher, Mimi Gold, who had been my first point of contact when I was told about the program. She erred with PaviElle instantly, because she treated her like a baby in the cafeteria. I observed that PaviElle was mad but I ignored the situation to prevent a scene. Her mood changed

On the day of the field trip PaviElle was happy and looking forward to the outing. As we got ready to leave the house she said, "Mom, I don't like Mimi."

I explained to her that it wasn't a good enough reason not to like her because she treated her like a baby. I told her Mimi was just meeting her for the first time and would learn soon. When I dropped her off at the center I saw Mimi and told her how PaviElle felt about her. She said she would step up her teaching and challenge her more. At the end of the trip you could see the joy on her face as she smiled from ear to ear, telling me the great time she had especially the trees and trains. She actually read a book before going to bed and was feeling less exhausted.

As the days of the program got into high gear her endurance got better but she had problems with the food at the center because of her being allergic to corn. Loretta came to the rescue and made sure there was the right food available for her to eat every day.

She began to complain about the new routine of her life and going up and down the stairs in physical therapy every day. I had to encourage her and explain the importance of the therapy to improve her balance and fears. I also told her that life in general is a routine for all, whether we are rich or poor. Her mood swings concerned me so I spoke with Loretta and she intervened and things got better. Her emotions were also very raw. She would look at her toes and cry so hard it broke my heart causing me to also break into tears. She told me maybe God had a reason for what happened at that later as she improved she also wanted to meet President Obama and his daughter Malia because she had allergies.

I wrote numerous letters to President Obama, First Lady Michelle Obama, Vice President Joe Biden, his wife, Dr. Biden, David Axelrod, advisor to the President, Valarie Jarrett advisor to the President, and Arnie Duncan, Education Secretary. The responses came in the way of form-letters or most times there was no response.

Finally, there was a response from President Obama's office by a message left on my home telephone's voice mail, something I had no time or desire to check. I am still wondering why they did not call my cell phone after not reaching me at home. When I did check I discovered a woman named Maude left the message and when I returned the call, she offered an invitation to come to the White House, but we had just one day to get to Washington which was impossible because of our situation at the time. I have been trying ever since, to get another date. When I pressed a staff member she informed me that policies are not made based on peoples personal issues like what happened to my daughter. I explained to her that I wanted to tell the president about our tragedy because he was at that time dealing with the healthcare reform issue, and I assumed our situation would have been relevant, because it was a hospital error that almost took my only child's life. She expressed sympathy and asked how my daughter was doing.

Later in December of 2009 she called again to invite us to the White House Christmas tree lighting ceremony, a White House traditional be possible. I thanked Maude and asked if she would keep trying because PaviElle was looking forward to meeting with him. She said she would see what was possible but up to this day we have not received a call to reschedule. I recently sent Maude an email and wrote several letters to President Obama with no response. PaviElle is extremely disappointed and insists I keep writing.

The Make a Wish Foundation managed to get PaviElle one of her wishes. She went through a number of rejections with her first choice Oprah Winfrey who we were told does not grant wishes. Then there was Tiger Dow but we learned that would take an extremely long time, and Venus and Serena Williams and Tyra Banks had problem with scheduling.

Finally, meeting Raven Simone was the only possibility, at a meeting at a concert in Georgia at Great Adventure Park. PaviElle enjoyed the meeting but it lasted only long enough for her to get an autograph. I appreciated the chance for her to meet Raven because she watched her on television for several years. I wanted to make it possible for children with illnesses to meet with their favorite celebrities in a more intimate setting for a long enough time so they can actually have a conversation with the celebrity. I embarked on my own campaign of meeting Oprah Winfrey but was unsuccessful after countless emails and letters.

But, back to PaviElle's struggles at recovery. There were days she would be both happy and sad. It felt like we were constantly on a roller coaster of emotions. Some days she made us laugh telling us her projected graduation day from the program would be February 29, 2008. I began to think the number 29 was somehow pivotal in our lives, but instead of the big negative of May 29, 2007, the date was now in a more positive way.

Some days PaviElle felt like herself again, although being faced with the grueling therapies and teaching to recapture her beautiful mind. Her visits to public places and stores were increasing rapidly, most of the time upon her requests. It was delightful for me to watch her blossom again and her wanting to go to familiar places, like Costco, TJ Maxx and Phipps Mall to visit her favorite candy store, Riverside Sweets.

After two weeks she was visibly stronger with better endurance and looking less like someone that was brain damaged and disabled. I felt good about the obvious progress, but sad for the other children and their families who were not having such great and rapid results. I prayed and counseled several parents and gave them words of encouragement and hope, showing them pictures of how PaviElle looked before she got to Atlanta. My action definitely gave the families hope and belief in miracles as they looked at the pictures and video that I shared. All the therapists were doing their best to move her along, and keep the pace of her recovery from stalling, so sometimes they pushed too hard like in physical therapy and when we got home her injured toe would be bleeding without them seeing.

The weekly field trips were very effective and stimulating for her brain, and as the weeks rolled on the journey seemed increasingly

During the absorption of my time and my total commitment to PaviElle's recovery, my close friends kept reminding me that I should be careful not to forget my husband and his male needs which meant his sexual needs. But, despite their subtle reminders, my mind was just not into sex, and I kept wondering how could they think I could even contemplate sex at such a disastrous and tragic time. My body was weak, my emotions were frazzled, my heart was broken and I felt like a fragile broken person who had to be strong, resilient and fight for the care and recovery of my child. "Am I wrong to feel so empty and broken?" I asked myself. There was no immediate answer so I continued to press onward in my mission and persevere. But, as it would turn out my friends promptings were in some way prophetic, as it was proven that men, regardless of how adverse the environment of their life may be, constantly crave sex.

It was now Christmas time, PaviElle's most loved holiday since she was a toddler. How would we celebrate Christmas 2007? At Thanksgiving it was great to give God thanks for all his blessings and for her speedy recovery. But what did she really need for Christmas? I asked her, but her list was very short, and no one in our family was feeling the spirit of the holidays.

We had several milestones to celebrate but we knew the road ahead would still be long and winding, with major potholes before we could really begin to enjoy the holidays again. However, Lloyd and I nonetheless got her gifts, and on Christmas Eve we put them out because she went to bed very early.
When Christmas Day arrived and she saw the gifts she was very

from truly getting what they deserved in a lawsuit because President George W. Bush had successfully capped the amounts they could claim in a suit. When laws like these are passed we as individuals do not pay attention because we never assume that a blazing fire involving DEADLY NEGLIGENCE can actually reach our house.

I began to think about what would President Bush and First Lady Laura Bush do if the patient who suffered from medical negligence was one of their beautiful twin girls, they had obviously struggled to have. My resentment for the legal system only grew as our legal journey for justice ensued.

After opening presents and having breakfast we ended the day having Christmas dinner at my Aunt Cislyn's house with lots of family members.

The worst year of my daughter's and my life was coming, thankfully, to an end. Deep in my heart and soul I could see the stress and worry my mother and my husband were experiencing. They in turn expressed their worry for me especially because of my significant weight loss, coupled with all the things I was forced to do for PaviElle because she was unable to do them for herself. However, I did not have time to dwell on personal condition because I was mother and it was my duty to support her, and much more, I loved her with all my heart.

Rehab pace at CHA was moving with great speed regardless of the holiday season and I made sure she did not miss a single day. The left so I was determined to prepare myself for the continued improvement in her health, happiness, well being, and succeed in all the legal battles that lay ahead that I knew had to be waged to right the wrong done to her. We quietly counted down the hours on New Year's Eve at my cousin Lee's apartment, and were led in a deeply spiritual prayer by Portia, another cousin. We watched the ball drop in New York's Time Square while playing games and reflecting on the major tsunami that had flooded our lives and created a disaster of unimaginable proportions. Then, within moments it was a new year and a new day and we were all happy.

We stayed in on New Year's Day and PaviElle was excited about going back to the rehab program that had become an integral part of her life, and another field trip that was planned for the movies. She again wanted an explanation for all the scars on her body and feet, for which I had to explain another heartbroken time. I felt very sad when I was faced with explaining to my beautiful daughter that her scars were there because of those idiot nurses and doctors at the hospital in Palm Beach who had almost ruined her life. All her hopes of becoming a dermatologist and restaurateur hung in an undetermined balance, like a dangling string of injustice while all we could do was wait for whatever uncertainties that lay ahead.

Lloyd had to return to Florida for work because there were still obligations to meet there. PaviElle was very sad at him going, but he tried successfully to explain as best he could. As I saw her in that state of melancholy my heart ached, and I again wondered how this tragedy happened and for the umpteenth time asked myself why did

Deadly Negligence **131**

to suffer the way we had. I thought of the scripture that God will turn your tragedy and make it for good but this was hard for me to imagine.

I started the next day to seek out the mothers who had children in the program and asked if they would be willing to speak on camera if I could succeed in producing a documentary about brain injuries. They all said a resounding. "Yes!" I then worked with the mother of one of the children, Eric, to share all the information I had found out about the sleeping pill Ambien and the results it had on individuals who had suffered a brain injury. She had someone in her family follow up and tried it with some visible results. Her next step was to dig deeper and got the doctors on board. I have continued with this effort, and also got other victims to believe in the power of prayers and miracles by sharing our story and creating a website. The site was done with the help of Mr. Bender and his friend John, with an anonymous donor who pays for maintaining the site on the Internet.

PaviElle right before she became ill

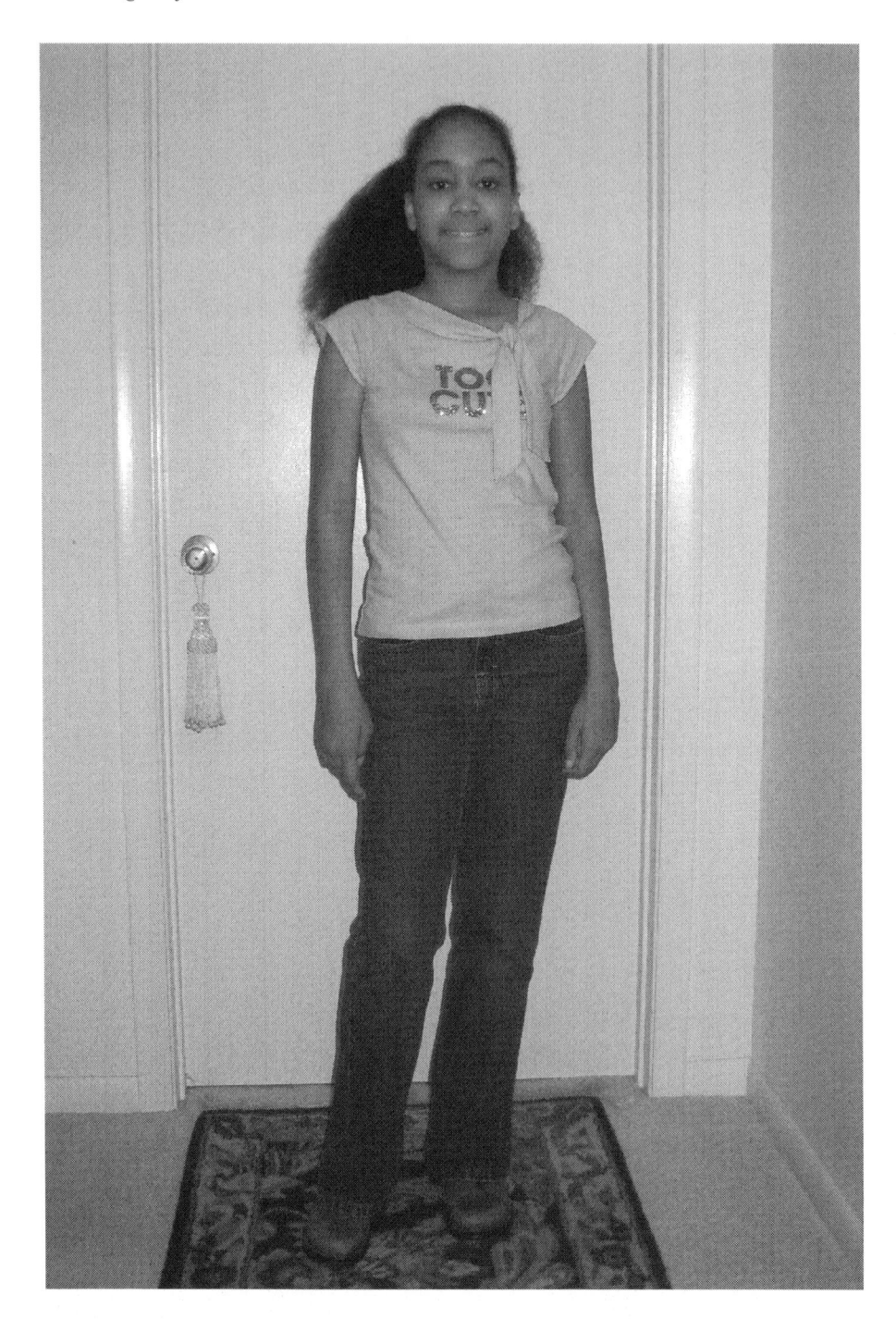

PaviElle during her recovery

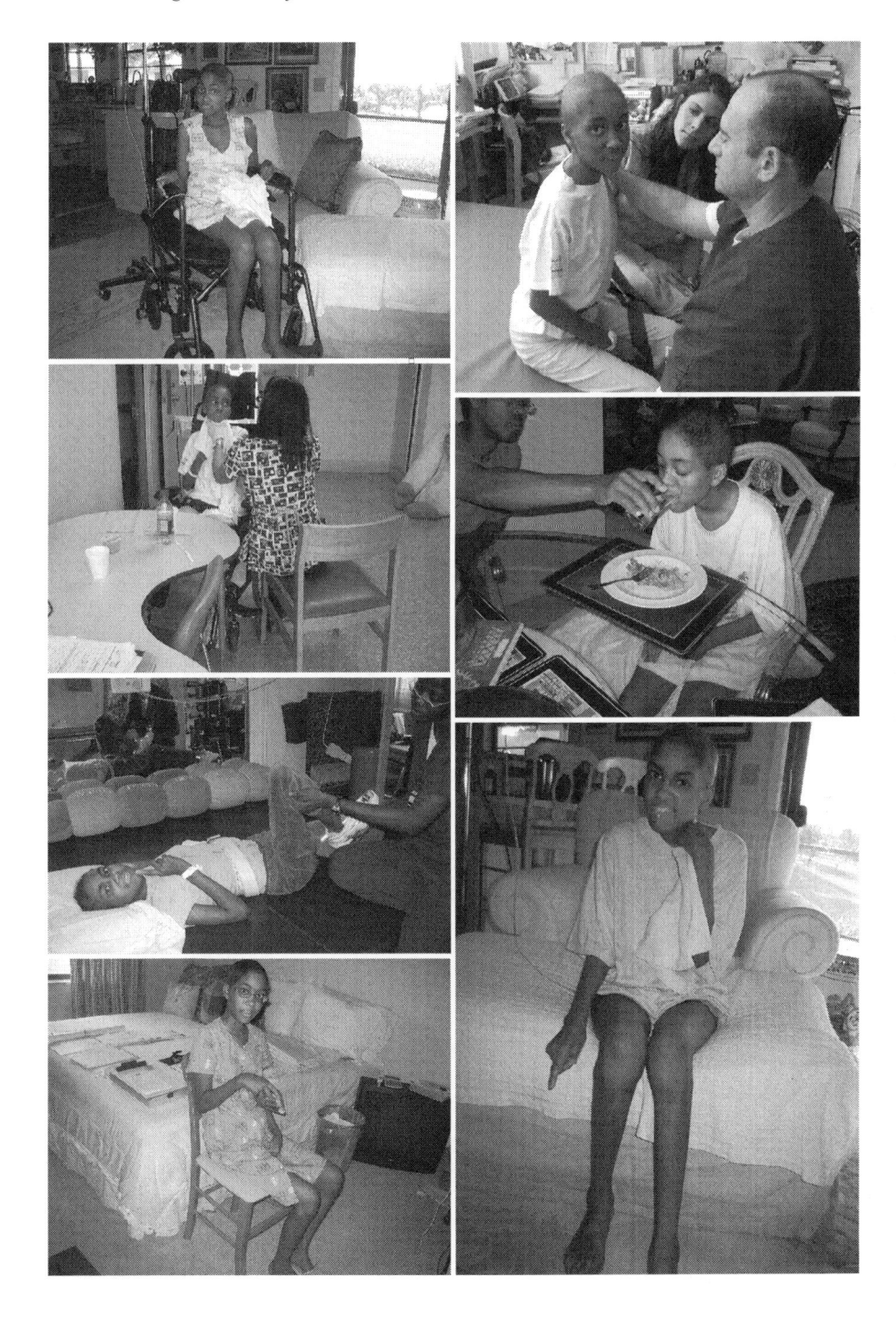

Chapter 11

he new year began with a request from the hospital's attorney for a list of all the things PaviElle could no longer do. I got to work and when Lloyd and I were on a conference call with our attorney Ron Rosen, we were ready to deliver. As I read the list my tears flowed and the hospital's lawyer became so overwhelmed that he said "Okay, Diana, never mind, I'll get a copy of the list from your attorney."

This telephone conversation and interview pained me deeply in my heart and soul. It gave me a glimpse of what was to come, as we forged into the legal genre of innuendoes and persecution by the hospital's legal team that even tried to blame me, and dug up my past medical history, to devise a claim of my perceived INSANITY.

As my sad mood persisted I was led by the Holy Spirit to read Jeremiah chapter 33, verse 3, and Jeremiah 30, verse 17. When I read both verses I was in awe that God had heard and answered my prayer. I shouted, "I love you God."

As PaviElle's slow recovery continued she managed to put a plastic

Deadly Negligence

I stood almost breathless the next morning when we got to the center watching her struggle with determination to hang her coat on the coat hook, remove the pen from the pocket and put her schedule in the folder. I quickly put on my sunglasses so neither she nor her teacher, Mimi, who was speaking to me about information she had requested from PaviElle's former school in Florida, could see my eyes filled with tears. I was so distressed with what I had just witnessed, but I congratulated PaviElle for her effort and she whispered in my ear, "I am okay mom you can go now."

I hustled to the car and broke down crying and screaming. An angel intervened when my cell phone rang. it was Mr. Bender who listened and gave me some encouraging words and prayer. After his call I thought about Prophetess Peart and gave her a call.

The tears continued to flow with my mind over laden with PaviElle's situation as I told Dr. Peart the core of my misery. I told her of seeing my sweet girl when all was well on March 19, 2007 when Dr. Namdoog said she was totally healed of JRA but she still needed to continue taking the medicine. I told her I adamantly disagreed with him and voiced my opinion. I related that I knew I should have listened to my inner voice and mother's intuition and stop giving her the medicine. I reflected on her great performance as the narrator of the Spanish end of year play and the scholarship she received from the college in Daytona to attend for the summer to learn about the transportation industry. I told her I had been asking God, over and over, "Why?" I also told Prophetess about how much we loved PaviElle cooking dinner for us before she became ill, and how worried I was that she supernatural God, a God of miracles and restoration who cures all diseases and sickness. I told both Prophetess and Mr. Bender that I was always on the 'God level of miracles' while everyone else was on the 'reality level.' Mr. Bender said God is still working miracles but because PaviElle made strides so quickly and at a fast pace it was similar to losing weight.

When you lose a lot of weight fast, you reach a plateau, but in the end when the lost weight is maintained you appreciate that all the sacrifice was worthwhile. After hearing me out, Prophetess said she would fast for PaviElle, then prayed with me and read Psalms 27 to me. She told me I could call her anytime, even at 4:00 a.m.

Although it had been a draining day, good news came when I picked PaviElle up later from the center. She was so thrilled to let me know that she was remembering how to do square roots, perimeter and other math problems. But her disappointment was also apparent when she told me her occupational therapist, Lisa, was moving to Las Vegas and another therapist, named Rachelle would be her primary replacement. She did not handle changes very well since this tragedy so I hoped for the best relationship between her and Rachelle.

Another field trip was coming so I was sure this would distract her from the looming change. Sadly, she found the trip to the Discovery Mills boring, but she improved a lot on hitting the golf ball. Everyone at the center kept asking me how I was doing and my response was always, "I'm good, but I do have dark days and nights." Although she was making progress it seemed very slow so I was feeling stretched her left hand more relaxed and when I held that hand she no longer screamed. She was more alert, taking out her own clothes, able to hold a bag and eat a Jamaican patty, use a large fork at dinner, and at bedtime she got in bed under the covers and pulled it over her face by herself. She watched Harry Potter movies on the Disney Network and remembered reading the first book in the series. As I watched her, despite my human impatience, I still marveled at God's goodness, and kept repeating, "God is Truly Great!!!!"

Amazingly, it began to snow in Atlanta and this was great for her memory. She ran outside and played in the snow as it came down, then coming back inside tried hard to take off her clothes and get into the shower. She then announced that she wanted a latte-coffee with whip cream on top from Starbucks. This was such a surprise and I had to remind her that she was only thirteen and drinking coffee was not allowed. However, to make her happy and stop her from constantly asking for the latte, I took her to a nearby Starbucks when the weather got better. She was very excited and enjoyed the experience.

Her left hand kept showing improvement but she was terrified of using the treadmill at the center, crying profusely when she was asked to go on it. Lavonda, her physical therapist tried unsuccessfully to talk her through her fear, but I managed to calm her and gave her confidence and things got better with the treadmill exercise. She was also having red spots on her skin because of her allergy to corn, so Loretta had to make sure she was not given anything to eat that had corn. She was beginning to sleep through the night and woke pertaining to the lawsuit against the hospital by telephone with my lawyer, Ron Rosen, Lloyd and the hospital's attorney. PaviElle sensed my anxiety and low feeling which I tried to keep inside, not wanting to worry my own mother. She asked me "Mom are you tired of me being sick?" Of course, I told her I was not.

The day that I had to give my unsworn statement was January 25, 2008. I was devastated because I had to retell the entire tragic story of what happened at the hospital when my child almost died because of negligence. Towards the end of the very long interview I was crushed, mad and cried all the way through to the end. When I hung up the telephone I felt like someone had literally ripped my heart out of my chest and I just could not stop crying. It was a good thing my room was upstairs and my mom being a little hard of hearing could not hear my bawling.

Amid all the success, improvement in PaviElle's toe on her left foot and her sharper memory she picked up the flu virus apparently from my mom who had some of the symptoms. I was beaten down because she already had so much to deal with and being ill with the flu would only cause her to miss days of intense rehab.

On the first day of absence from rehab she said she missed Florida, started crying, saying she wanted to go back home to her room and more familiar surroundings. I went into extreme high gear to give her all the homemade remedies, from chicken soup to Vicks Vapor Rub. Dr. Rubin recommended tenting - a remedy for clearing her nose, using tea trash, orange peel, with hot water in a sink and necessary to prolong the program. The weekly and monthly process of waiting to be told if Medicaid would pay for the program was absolutely nerve racking and causing me to have heart palpitations. Each time an approval call came I would have moments of celebration, but reminded myself it could all come to an end suddenly.

As the end of January approached the highlights were that Dr. Rubin was coming to visit PaviElle, and Lloyd would be returning from Florida, but she continued to cry wanting to go back home to Florida. I didn't know what to do. Asking God for His help and direction was my only option because she was obviously stressed and wanted me to grant her the wish to go back home. I knew she loved Atlanta so I was confused about what she was feeling. When Dr. Rubin and her dad arrived she calmed down somewhat, as they explained everything to her about why we had to move to Atlanta and the necessity for being in the intense therapy program at CHA.

She was now in the final month of therapy and the center moved to a new location that was long in the making. With this move I hoped that she would be approved for another month in March, because the success was so real. She was enjoying the field trips increasingly, laying out her clothes from the night before, undressing herself to get in the shower and turn the water on, although her left hand was still not functioning well. She tried to make her bed, blew bubbles, and slept in her own bed by herself all night long. Unfortunately, she broke out in hives after eating peanut butter at the center, and was itching so badly she wanted to sleep with me. It was a move backwards, but I allowed her to do so, trying anything to make her proportion. I had to rush home and bring new clothes and towels. She was so embarrassed, cried very hard, and kept apologizing to her grandma saying, "I'm sorry grandma." Mom and I took a very long time to convince her it was all okay and that she had done nothing

A field trip was organized to go to the University of Georgia for a fundraiser but PaviElle refused to attend unless Loretta was going. She being very stubborn so eventually Loretta went and they had a great time. The trip must have triggered something with her memory because when she got home she asked to borrow my cell phone. She scrolled through the files and found a recording she had made a long time ago when she was calling her dad to come and cut a mango. She then tried to wash a cup and plate using her right hand only and took a shower, dried herself and got out of the stall by herself. I stood there staring and shouted, "What a mighty God we serve. This is a great thing, Thank you God." She was working really hard at rehab but her limitations continued to make me sad. In the final month at rehab PaviElle announced she found a new friend. She also still wanted to go home and said she needed to have a television hanging from the ceiling in her bedroom, a walk in closet with a turnstile so that her clothes would be easily accessible, a sitting area to hang out, a shower seat and two golf carts parked in the garage. Another announcement was, "Mom, I'm happy, but sad, because Mimi told me I am not ready to go back to school if we move back to Florida but would have to continue with homebound school."

Her thoughtful requests and emotions surprised me, causing me to was fantastic and revived her memory of going to the circus when she was much younger. She also recognized someone in the crowd that we had not seen for a very long time and was happy to say hello. This I thought was great because it also depicted her confidence about her appearance and the loss of her long hair.

I was beginning to see several programs on CNN Nightline and other networks about hospital negligence and medication that were harming individuals. This made me mad, thinking how ironic it was that all these unfortunate events were taking place around the country including with movie stars. I resented the fact that the stars were being featured on television and ordinary people like my daughter and other families had no voice nor anyone to speak for them.

February 19, 2008 became a significant date when I received a package after I dropped PaviElle at rehab. It was discharge paperwork that I was required to sign whether I agreed with the decision to discharge her from the therapy program, or not.

I kept the document for a few days as I questioned why Medicaid would not pay, and pondered on the benefits she would lose because of their refusal. I was counseled by the director, therapists and staff at the rehab center that returning home to Florida would be the best and most progressive for PaviElle. They said it was better for her to be in familiar surroundings of home and out-patient therapy, where the results would be great based on their experience. When I picked her up that day from rehab, she asked me to call everyone in Florida serious, so I asked Dr. Rubin if she could possible plan a welcome event. She agreed, saying it would be no problem, that she would make all the arrangements for a welcome-home party.

As the days went by leading to graduation from the program PaviElle kept insisting on having the welcome-home party. At this juncture she was working extremely hard especially on her left hand. I cried out to God and called on the belief in my faith, as I knew for sure she would be totally healed, restored and cured in every way. I shared my belief with her and together we believed, as the scripture says, *"If two of you shall agree on earth as touching, anything that they shall ask it shall be done for them of my father which is in heaven."* - Matthew chapter 18 verse 19.

She began to count down the days when her graduation would take place from the program and her final trip to the center would be a reality. She seemed so thoughtful and precise about her needs and wants that this made me skeptical and happy at the same time. She was joking around saying she wanted us to start walking home. We had a good laugh together; wishing home was Santa Barbara in California, my favorite place in all America.

The rash she had disappeared and we were elated about this. However, even with the great mood she was in, the flu was still trying to knock her down and I was trying to do everything I could possible do to prevent it from affecting her. I eventually succeeded in having her rid of the flu symptoms by using home remedies and over the counter drugs, in association with lots of rest and drinking plenty of seen the obvious improvements she was making. I asked numerous questions and did my own research in an attempt to refute what they were telling me about the lack of any real benefit if she remained in the program for one more month. Under duress I realized my choices were zero and fighting Medicaid to pay for the extra month would prove futile, so I reluctantly surrendered my efforts to resist and signed the documents.

Two days before her final day at the rehab center PaviElle had to stay home because she wasn't feeling great as fighting the flu was still a big challenge. Our desire to go home was overtaking all our thoughts and I decided to call Prophetess for some support. She prayed with me and read John chapter 14 verses 13 and 14: *"And whatsoever ye shall ask in my name, that will I do, that the Father may be glorified in the son. If ye shall ask any thing in my name,* I will do it."
I felt revived and good, but told her, "With the sudden brain damage of our perfect child, the shock, struggle and devastation is very hard." She gave me more encouraging words as always, and my heart pounded with a little more hope after hearing her voice.

PaviElle managed to find enough energy to go to rehab the day before her final day and graduation, staying all day. Lloyd arrived that day so her spirits were lifted enough for her to invoke humor, asking me, "Mom will there be a welcoming committee when I get back to Florida?"

Her question reminded me to call Dr. Rubin about the welcoming arrangements she had promised to look about and she told me not working with PaviElle and praised her for her determination. They expressed to me that they knew I was disappointed she was not allowed to stay in the program for another month but said I would see positive results ahead. They also thanked me for the support I was giving my daughter and assured me that was more important than another month in the program.

PaviElle received rave reviews at the graduation ceremony and everyone was hopeful for more improvement when she returned to familiar territory in Florida, where her injury occurred. Prizes and surprises and lots of photographs and videos were part of the graduation ceremony which had each graduate wearing a gold cap and gown. As a family we felt various emotions: apprehension, sadness, joy and shed tears, but in my heart and soul I felt jilted out of another month of therapy that I had convinced myself would have greater results. I was indeed thankful for the months that Medicaid had paid for Rehab, and again was grateful and also thankful to God for the progress she had made because of the intense treatment she did receive at that incredible facility.

The graduation ceremony was really a good one and PaviElle had a super-day, but she kept pressing, asking, "Mom, am I just going home without celebration when I arrive?" I wanted to appease her curiosity but I was committed to keeping the secret that Dr. Rubin and Ms. Stover, her past language arts teacher, were planning a great surprise, although it was not a party. I honestly did not know the details either so I really had no information to share that could ruin the surprise.

since I was aware that she would have to restart out-patient therapy on our return to Florida, I took advantage of the delay to call APS and contact all her former therapists so that there would be no time wasting in the continuation of her therapies.

Chapter 12

he day we chose to return to Florida was one that is etched in my memory, and I am sure of PaviElle's and Lloyd. My mom was the only one who was sad about our departure. It was a bright, sunny, gorgeous day filled with beautiful white clouds encased in the brilliant blue sky, and to top that, PaviElle was feeling much better. I feared the long ride to Florida would have made her totally exhausted, but although she was excited to move back home she slept almost the entire journey.

It was late when we got home, but in the dark she could see the huge bunch of balloons tied to our mailbox with a seemingly endlessly long banner that read, "WELCOME HOME PAVI, WE ALL LOVE YOU." She screamed so loud with excitement and joy that I actually jumped. We called Dr. Rubin immediately and expressed our profound thanks. As we got closer to our front door we saw there were several gifts and tokens from her friends and teachers stacked by the door. I kept thanking Dr. Rubin telling her what a blessing she was to our family. The atmosphere was filled with happiness, joy and laughter as I watched her relish in the love and thoughtfulness shown to her by her classmates and teachers.

and determination. Getting back into the routine of rehab at APS was stressful because space was limited for all the therapies. My thoughts were constantly in overdrive and I felt as if my life was a total wreck. I cannot relate how many times I poised the question, "God, why is this happening to my sweet child? She has never hurt or harmed anyone."

Malissa advised me to let PaviElle use the computer as much as possible, and Nicole was impressed by the improvement of her hand writing. We acted immediately on Malissa's advice and the result was fantastic. Malissa also told me to buy the Vivaldi Four Seasons CD and play it for PaviElle as often as possible with her using a headphone. She said the positive results of brain injury patients to music were difficult to explain, but insisted I tried having Pavi play the CD.

Obviously, I bought the CD and it absolutely worked in several ways. PaviElle seemed more alert and focused, remembering more things about her life and figured out how to play all her computer games that she struggled to remember especially her favorite, Roller Coaster.

Moving back to Florida had challenges because we had lost our consistent spots for each therapy; doctors had to be reenlisted, a new homebound teacher had to be assigned so she could get prepared for reentering middle school. However, the greatest challenge laid at home.

Lloyd had embarked upon remodeling of our bathrooms without much help. I thought what he was doing was admirable but he failed which made me feel even more uncomfortable. At the risk of hurting his feelings, I decided to add to a list of things that I had to accomplish in the urgency of getting the renovations completed so that I would not have to continue living in a dusty, uncomfortable, disorganized, unusable construction zone. At the same time I did not want to appear ungrateful to my husband because he was obviously trying to finish a task he started in good faith.

It is my nature to get things started and completed within the shortest possible time, because procrastination, excuses, and the words, "I can't." are topics I have absolutely no tolerance for. Therefore I did my best to control the dust, and hired workmen to help so the project was placed on the fast track to completion.

At nights Lloyd was constantly falling asleep in the living room after he ate dinner; usually in front of the television. This practice infuriated me and only helped to create a contentious home life, on top of the challenges of PaviElle's illness that I had to deal with and had so deeply affected our lives. At the time I was not aware that Lloyd was being unfaithful, so PaviElle and I took the home situation in stride. When he fell asleep we would do fun things to jog her memory like trying to open her diary that she had locked and could not remember the password. Eventually when it was busted open we learned the password was "punk rocker," something that was not even on any of our minds because that was so contrary to her personality.

On opening the diary it brought back her memory to the extent that she could explain to me why she had chosen the password. She said

Deadly Negligence

about small things like the misplaced remote control, and he would storm off, shower and go to bed. Following one particular incident with the remote he left for work without even saying goodbye, and didn't bother calling the entire day to check on PaviElle, and totally refused to speak to me. This behavior was unusual, but I would later find out why. My daughter and I noticed how mean and argumentative and even hostile he had become but made a decision to ignore the situation until it became unbearable. He would barely say hello when he got home, and one evening I decided to ask what was the problem and he replied, "Pigs don't speak."

I was puzzled by his response, but immediately recalled then that one evening when he was screaming and shouting at me with looks of hate, that I did tell him he was behaving like a pig. I told him that because he had become and behaved like someone we did not recognize. He seemed like a stranger and later I would find out that I was actually sleeping with the enemy. I told myself that taking care of PaviElle was much more important than poking around and checking upon him to find out if he had another woman. So, I pressed on with all my duties and responsibilities knowing that God would send the answer to me if I simply trust Him. I also noticed he was coming home later and later every evening, with excuses that just did not make sense even though he was self employed at the time. I was just not buying the explanations. Always trust your intuition and instincts even when you are occupied with more urgent situations.

On March 12, 2008 after Lloyd continued with his malice, and refused to speak to me, I decided to call him on his cell phone. I asked him a relationship with another woman, but I had no proof or time to confront the issue. I continued the conversation asking him, "If you were away for months, and came back to a house you left in order and found both bathrooms in a state of disrepair, dust and chaos, your favorite plants dead from lack of water, your car not serviced with the gas tank on empty, what would you do, how would you feel and how would you have reacted?"

He replied, "You think you are always right, Mrs. McLaughlin." I was so mad I called his sister Sharon and replayed the conversation for her so she could spare me from the thought that I was going crazy. She very calmly said, "He really should have finished the bathrooms, even one."

I said thanks and got back to all I needed to accomplish that day. I later called Lloyd about getting a back-pack for PaviElle, he responded in the same cold manner. He actually came home just before the scheduled visit of the new homebound teacher to get something from the garage and he did not even bother to come into the house to check on us or meet Grady, the teacher, who arrived while he was outside in the garage. I was flabbergasted, but kept my cool and tried to camouflage my outrage from PaviElle.

Although he was not speaking to me and being so distant to us I continued to do marketing for his company. I met a man, Frank, at the center who was a developer in Palm Beach County, who also constructed buildings in the Dominican Republic. I told him about my husband's electrical company and his qualifications so he gave

Deadly Negligence 151

therapy for PaviElle free. I called and spoke to a man named Mike who was unable to help but gave me another name, Randy, a woman. She was wonderful and full of compassion when she heard what had happened to my daughter. She promised to find me help and called back with information regarding the ELKS organization. However, it was not for speech, but rather occupational therapy, which turned out to be our good fortune. Teri, an expert occupational therapist then came into our lives. She is still with us treating PaviElle until this day and she was another miracle. She helped us receive the speech therapy that we were seeking originally. God bless the ELKS organization they have been a savior.

After a very long, frustrating process, the renovation of the bathroom was completed and our home returned to a dust free and organized environment once again. It was truly a cause for celebration when the last row of gorgeous glass subway tiles were installed in my daughter's bathroom. It was really a thrill to have the house looking so orderly again.

When PaviElle met the new homebound teacher, Grady, she liked her although she was cautious and somewhat resistant at first, but eventually they both worked together beautifully. We also continued to visit Dr. Rubin who would help with teaching her science, math, Spanish and Italian and make delicious Jewish specialties like turkey and cheese patties with cucumber salad. She educated us about her culture and told stories of her childhood and adult life. We would sit outside and enjoy the beautiful lake watching the jet skiers go by and enjoy the beauty of her backyard. This ritual became something

God for placing her in our lives at Okeeheelee Middle school where PaviElle had been a student. She not only helped with relearning skills and information, but legal matters including giving a deposition about the girl she knew before the tragedy and was willing to testify for us if the lawsuit went to court. "Anything for Pavi," she would always say and, "Don't worry Diana, I will attend Pavi's graduation and her wedding; you'll see."

She gave me information about colleges in Europe that are actually American schools and those in the United States that would work for PaviElle later in her school years. I took all the information she gave me and researched them so when the time came I would be armed for whatever battle that was ahead. It seemed PaviElle's tragedy had made me more deeply involved in research because sometimes the information I found became a life saver for her. Mr. Bender was also consistent in helping her with reading and comprehension, prayer and encouragement.

At that point of her recovery it struck me that it was very strange that all the friends I had who used to call me almost every day to tell their personal stories, or asked for advise no longer called, and all the friends who had promised so faithfully to help me with PaviElle's care when we left the hospital reneged on this promise. The only genuine offer I received was from a nurse named Pat whom we met at Jackson Memorial. I later found out that we had mutual friends and I also knew some of her cousins, Monica and Joan. Pat lived all the way in Pembroke Pines, a hour and a half away from my house but she came and visited us, read and talked to PaviElle for a long

PaviElle looked and how fast she was recovering. Judy, who remained a dear friend, would call and ask if I needed anything and brought clean white towels that I was using each day for Pavi's care. The towels became a life saver and saved me from doing laundry every day.

As PaviElle progressed with the various therapies she began reaching more milestones like putting on her seat belt, locking and opening it, but would become frustrated some days, declaring, "I am tired of this crap."

I had to take time out to explain the importance of therapy that would help her regain full use of her left hand, have clear speech, and balance on and ride her bike again. These talks got no easier for me and kept reminding me of what she was going through and all she had to endure at such a young age. Fortunately for me her frustrations never lasted very long because she had to a great extent retained her happy and easy personality that everyone had cautioned me that she might lose because of the brain injury.

We were at a crossroad with the problem with her left hand because nothing was really working. Dr. Podda her hematologist/oncologist called from Jackson Memorial to check on her progress and suggested the success of Botox and the possibility of using it to treat her left hand. He knew I would research it so he laughed and told me to call him when I made my decision. I not only researched Botox but sought the advice of Dr. Lue, her Neurologist; Malissa, the speech therapist; and Teri, the occupational therapist. They all agreed Botox faith in his supernatural healing powers. I had heard of the success of Botox in removing the wrinkles in the faces of some women, but also learned that one of the side effects was that the part of the face injected would no longer move. I was confident about my decision. Dr. Lue had told me, when I asked him about using the drug, that he too would give it thought until her next appointment and if he thought it would be beneficial and if I agreed he would give PaviElle the injection at his office.

When we next saw him he said he was not convinced either that it would help her with the movement and use of the left hand. Therefore he also made the decision to not give the Botox injection. As I continued to muddle through the maze of therapy, paperwork, research, trying to get accurate information about the right school to accommodate my child, who now had the label of being 'Brain Damaged and Disabled,' the world began to seem so cruel and daunting. Everyone tried to tell me what my child could or could not do, placing limitations on her abilities and wanted to place her with other great children who had other labels like Retarded, Autistic and other learning disabilities. I thought when my mother worked with the State of New York with children who were disabled because of various circumstances the key word was INCLUSION into the regular population.

It was mind boggling, frustrating, and depressing to see the EXCLUSION and the fight a parent had to be prepared for, if, like me, they wanted their child to be restored and achieve the success they once had. Life is sure bitter sweet. I did what I knew best, throwing my daughter, was really relevant as Jill had experienced the same fate; the only difference was that PaviElle's experience resulted from medical negligence.

Before I embarked on the battle with the school choice for PaviElle, a battle that would consume my days and nights, causing my brain to go into overdrive mode, I would be shaken to the core of my being, which made me to feel like I was walking on quicksand, sinking slowly into a nervous breakdown with no visible light at the end of the tunnel. I experienced a depth of indescribable emotions that had the power to take me down, were it not for God.

What might this be you ask? What was it that could destroy everything I believed to be true and honest during the absolute worst time of my entire life. I trusted that my husband, who I loved with all my heart and soul, would have taken the tragic journey with me like he pretended to, without throwing me to the wolves of distrust, disappointment and embarrassment.

Chapter 13

t was March 14, 2008 and my world was about to come crashing down like a bolt of lightning with the ability to kill. I woke up very early with a deep hole in my spirit and I knew when feelings of this kind gripped me there would be bad news from somewhere.

Early that morning I called BAK middle school in Palm Beach County based on the recommendation of the quality of their program for children with disabilities. As usual, I was passed on to several people before speaking with Susan Stevens, the ESE coordinator. After listening to my story and dilemma she informed me that the audition process had passed but I should call Mary Vreland because she was the one with the power to override the audition date and allow my child to have a chance of being admitted. I then called and spoke to one Debbie who had to find out if Mary would be able to speak with me and she promised to call me back. In this case, Mary was too important to speak with an average parent like me. These words were not said, but were implied. This reminded me of a conversation I had with a female who answered the telephone at the office of US Education Secretary Arnie Duncan, and who very firmly informed me when I asked to speak to the secretary, that Mr. Duncan does

Deadly Negligence **157**

message I left on her voice mail. I am sorry to inform you if you are, thankfully, reading this book you are on your own when you seek help from the government, and some public and private entities, but you must never give up. If one avenue fails, try another until someone hears your voice and your plea to help and protect your children. I also learned if your child is a smart student there were numerous opportunities and programs to reward that child. If you are poor and failing there are programs buried so deep in a sea that if you are unable to swim you are most certain to drown. If you find yourself with a child who is somewhere in the middle there are absolutely no programs, no help, and you will be fighting solo until God sends you an angel. Believe it or not there are still some in this failed education system in America.

On this day, the moment I spoke of earlier was about to hit me with a huge block used in making a solid house. My cell phone rang at exactly 9:31a.m. as I was having a conversation with Janet the physical therapist about PaviElle's progress and plans for the next week. The number came up as 'unknown' and usually I would not answer the call but my small internal voice, which is called the SPIRIT, spoke to me and said answer the call and ask the person to hold until you finished the conversation with Janet. I obeyed my inner voice. I got PaviElle ready, got into my Jeep and reengaged the female voice waiting on the cell phone. Immediately, without introduction, this woman declared, "Lloyd has a light skin long hair woman in her forties, who lives in Fort Lauderdale, and you should protect yourself from disease."

I said, "Why would I not, believe you?"

She said she did not know me personally but had seen me on television in Jamaica, and listened to me on the radio. She then proceeded to describe Lloyd. "He is an electrician, slim, wears glasses, has a grey Jeep, a white Jeep and a white truck and has even slept at her house overnight."

In receiving all this detailed information I just allowed her to continue talking because my daughter was in the Jeep so my tongue had to be tied and my feelings and emotions kept inside. The call continued until I got into my garage because she would not stop. I started to wonder if the woman she was telling me about was herself, but it could not be. I realized that she was using this call to avenge her own pain and suffering that she experienced with her own husband's infidelity so I continued to listen. Sensing that I had gotten to my destination she said goodbye, and wished me well hoping that I did not contract any disease or infection from my husband. I politely thanked her for the information and when she hung up I rechecked the screen of the phone to see if my eyes had deceived me but the number was indeed unknown.

At the end of that unbelievable call it struck me the woman on the other end of the phone sounded intensely wounded to her core, but she also left me with a wound that was filled with disgusting yellow puss that was bound to bleed when it got busted open, causing a scar that may never heal with an even scab.
My heart was about to burst out of my chest and seeing Lloyd's car

Deadly Negligence

are seeing a light skin, long hair, woman in her forties who lives in Fort Lauderdale and I should protect myself from disease. She also described you as an electrician, slim, wears glasses, has a grey jeep, white jeep and white truck and has even slept at the woman's house overnight. Is this true?"

He answered with the big lie, "Not me."

I opened the door as he told me the blatant lie, went to the master bedroom to use the bathroom to release the nervous stomach I had from hearing the news. When I finished I went to the kitchen where he was now sitting perched on a counter chair, and said to him, "Please remember I am a broadcaster and journalist. Tell me the truth now because you know I will investigate and find the truth."

The nervousness on his face was blinding and the lie seemed to have gobbled him up. I made another statement, "I hope you used a condom because if you brought home her disease to me I will kill you."

He immediately started to confess telling me the woman's name, phone number and address, when and how they met, who seduced whom, kept calling whom and, also another lie that he did use a condom. I also told him that I would not keep this a secret but I would call all his family and our friends who believed he was so wonderful as a husband giving complete support at this tragic time but he was out screwing around while PaviElle laid in the hospital near death. I knew my words would sting, as I reminded him that

He had no response. The fast pace of my brain knew that the most dangerous words in that call from the anonymous woman was disease. It kept racing through my thoughts what if this woman had AIDS or any other sexually transmitted disease?

It was Friday, and I knew getting an urgent appointment to see my OBGYN was impossible but I wasted no time and called her office anyway. The lady who answered asked me why I needed an immediate appointment when I had recently done my annual checkup with the doctor, so I told her what I had just found out about my husband's infidelity. She said, "I am so sorry," and gave me an appointment for early Monday morning. She also explained that the doctor would have me do an AIDS test, plus other tests, but not to worry because the place to do the test was in the same building, and all could be done the same day.

My next step was to carry out my threat of calling everyone. My first call was to my mom who I knew loved Lloyd dearly as a son-in-law. I barely said hello and she knew something devastating had happened. At first I could not get the words out as she asked, "What's wrong, did something happen to PaviElle."

To stop her anxiety, as I sat on the toilet, the words finally came out in a whisper, "I just got a call that Lloyd is sleeping with another

My mom was speechless and in a state of shock and disbelief. She knew that I always told Lloyd that when he found someone else he should simply call me and I would put his belongings at the door so thinking about the possible results of the various tests I must take on Monday.

Calling his cousin Yvonne in Tampa was difficult because I knew she adored him and thought we were such a great couple. She counseled me when I told the story and gave me her long story of infidelity with her own husband and the struggles she also had. She asked me to forgive Lloyd and stay in my marriage and promised that things would get better and back to normal but it would take a long time to be restored. Yvonne was a good supporter of PaviElle's recovery and was one of the family members who drove all the way from Tampa to Miami to visit my daughter while she was in Jackson Memorial hospital. I told her thanks for her kind words and for listening to my problems. She assured me that I could call her anytime day or night no matter how late it was.

I then called his sister Sharon but had to leave a voice mail and wait for a call back. She called me back quickly because she was mindful of her niece's illness. When she called her voice had a sense of panic but as I told her the story she got mad and refused to speak to her brother. I also called the number Lloyd had given me for his mistress, using his cell phone, but got her voice mail. I wanted to ask her directly if they had used a condom during their sexual escapades because I knew for sure he was lying.

We were scheduled to visit Sharon and her family because when they visited PaviElle she had just come out of the hospital and the visit was very traumatic for her sons Jason and Jarrett, so I wanted them course thinking it was him, informing him she would have to call back because Ms. Important was in a meeting. She heard me in the background so she knew their sordid affair was out in the light and I knew everything. Obviously, she did not have the guts or nerve to call back so I called her again with his phone when we arrived at Sharon's house. She answered, so I took Lloyd and Sharon into the bathroom, locked the door and put the phone on speaker and made him say hello to her. When I asked her if they used a condom when my husband screwed her, she said, "I don't play that. No condom was ever used."

He was stunned when she said that and went on to give her version of the story about how he had done electrical work for her and kept trying to hit on her, as if he badly wanted a woman. Her story continued as she said her ex-husband cheated on her and she told herself that if she had a relationship with a married man and the wife called she would speak the truth and tell the whole story.

My sister-in-law jumped in when this woman began to attack me about raising my voice and using profanity, instead of us having a civil conversation. Sharon shouted at her and asked how she could be talking about a civil conversation when she was sleeping with my husband. The heated conversation continued for a very long time and she pretended not to know who I was but later was forced to recant after she made a comment that confirmed she was lying. The rawness of the conversation continued as Lloyd kept asking her to confirm the things he was telling me and she laughed at him and really did not respond. She wanted me to have a civil conversation brother, venting her feelings of disappointment and disgust. When Paul, Sharon's husband got home I filled him in with all the details.

We left her house without resolution or comfort to go to Robbie's Restaurant to buy some jerk pork and chicken. I made my next call to Joan, my best friend at the time, giving her all the gory details and she was in a state of disbelief and shock. Before we got home we stopped to get something for PaviElle to eat and when Lloyd got out of the car she said, "Look at him, looking so innocent." I almost peed in my pants but asked her what she was talking about. She said, "I know things and, you know Mom, I'm entitled to know what's going on around here. I heard when you told him to close the door and don't let me see him bawling." I was so surprised at this I just said nothing.

I next called my other friend, Judy, and she kept saying she found it strange that he never came by her house to eat with them when PaviElle and I were in Atlanta, because we were all close friends. When we got home I forced him to call his brother Wayne in Jamaica, so I could give him the full story. Wayne asked to speak to him, but first asked me to try and work it out. Tony, his cousin in Orlando called and I did not hesitate to fill him in. He kept saying, "I thought Lloyd told me he does not do those things because his marriage is so good. I often use you guys as an example of a good marriage."

I also called Roberta my neighbor who filled in some of the areas he denied about sleeping overnight at his woman's house.
It was now, "Bawling Saturday." I was feeling pretty lousy, unable to

I would stay and continue to love him unconditionally, but would need time to sort things out. I told her that she must be insane to think I would do that, and emphasized that would not happen. She kept insisting, telling me I had to do it.

Eventually, I relented, and when we ended our call I went to Lloyd to tell him we needed to talk. He listened to me then hugged me and said thanks. I tried to be good, and even be nice to him but it was extremely difficult.

PaviElle and I left the house to visit Dr. Rubin because it was Saturday and this was part of our routine on the road to recovery. I was miserable, my mind kept going elsewhere and back to the disgusting actions of my husband. I tried so hard, but the nightmare continued to haunt me like I was in a ghost filled environment fighting to find my way to escape the torment and torture. The visit went well for PaviElle, but I felt so empty and was unable to share my devastation with Dr. Rubin because I did not want the visit to be about my sordid situation when it should be about my daughter. I sucked it up, but when we got home my cousin Simone called to see how we were

As I sat in the home office pondering and wallowing in my sorrow I had to tell Simone what Lloyd had done and she was mad. We talked for a very long time, and all of a sudden I broke down and began screaming out of control so loud that Lloyd came running into the office to see what had happened. He tried to console me, but I was hurting so bad. PaviElle also came in hugged, kissed me and begged road and cried buckets of tears, screamed and hollered.

It did not take long for PaviElle to realize that I was gone so she woke Lloyd up and he kept calling my cell-phone franticly. I did not answer. He got in his Jeep and drove around the neighborhood trying to find me. I could see him as he drove by but he could not see me. I decided to finally answer his call because I was concerned that he might have left PaviElle in the house by herself. He begged me to come back home but I was crying so hard he said he could not understand what I was saying.

Eventually at 3:00 a.m. I went back to the house while he was still on the phone talking to me. He was so obviously glad to see me. Back in our room I kept asking him when did he find time to have sex with his woman. He refused to answer, but I was relentless in my interrogation. Eventually he said it was once, one afternoon before he went on an appointment. I didn't believe a word of what he was telling me and kept asking him what kind of woman allows a man to have sex with her after having only one conversation with him, and worse, as I learned, with her teenage daughter living in her house. I told him she must have felt very bad about herself and have such low self esteem that no man wanted her, or she sleeps with all the workmen that does work for her at her house. I also asked him how he got the condom he claimed he used, but which she had disputed. He lied again, saying he left and went to the store to buy it. I then tried to get more intimate details, and asked him if the oral sex he got was that good that he was forced to go buy condoms to return to the woman for sexual intercourse. I was totally amazed at his lies, told me a story about his friend whose wife was ill and another woman who was a friend and had comforted him. First, according to Blue, the relationship was innocent, but then after a while it led into an intimate relationship that ruined his marriage. He tried to explain to me that Lloyd was a good guy and probably got caught up in the similar situation. He offered to speak with Lloyd, and said he would give me his support whenever I needed it. I thanked him for listening, and he said I could call him anytime.

I kept asking Lloyd more questions about his woman and pointed to her lies about not knowing me from radio and television and how she decided to sleep with married men because her husband cheated on her. I was also asking myself what was I going to do about the situation. Lloyd kept telling me he only had sex with this woman one time, but she insisted they had a relationship. I asked if he had kissed her and he said no. I did not believe anything he said. How would I get pass this I wondered. I had so much faith and trust in my husband, but it went down the drain in one sex moment. Why was my life so destroyed? I felt like I was being buried alive with my head barely above ground with many scary creatures lurking around me. I was deeply hurt by what Lloyd did and I wanted details, so I decided I had no choice but to call the woman and get her full side of the story in a calm and civil manner. However, I decided to wait until after my visit to the OBGYN.

On Monday, after a weekend that seemed like it would never end, I prepared to make the visit to OBGYN. Lloyd, remarkably, decided to go with me to the doctor because he knew PaviElle would be with

Deadly Negligence

for the doctor. When she arrived, she started the exam and asked why I was coming to see her so soon after my annual physical. I felt so ashamed and vulnerable as I told her the story. She gave me the utmost compassion and her wise counsel and took all the necessary body samples she needed for the AIDS test and for other sexually transmitted diseases. I was instructed where to go for more AIDS test upstairs. When I got there the room was filled with various types of individuals getting tested for different things. As I waited my thoughts were consumed with what the result would be and how many people in the room were experiencing my sordid predicament.

When the examiner called my name I quickly went in and I was given my instructions. As I laid there my life flashed before my face as the woman drew my blood. To relax me she began talking and asked the dreaded question, "Why are you doing the test?"

I was again forced to tell my heart wrenching story. She chuckled, then laced into her disgust for men who did not use condoms especially when they decided to cheat on their wives. She assured me that I was not alone because she had to do the tests for several women with my story every day. Observing my visible fear she made a decision to tell me right there and then that the HIV test was negative, but my doctor would call me with the results of the other STD tests. I expressed my eternal gratitude to her because she had spared me the anxiety and stress of waiting for the results even though there were other results to receive. I was content to get the results of the one test I was most concerned about. I felt as if I was spared a death sentence which I knew would only complicate my daughter's recovery. I left negative HIV test, but the bad news was that I had a vaginal infection that needed immediate treatment. She asked for the telephone number of my pharmacy, and said she would call in a prescription and I should go pick it up and begin using it right away. After our conversation I told Lloyd about the infection, and that he needed to be tested because he had infected me. Hearing this, his face turned white like a sheet, his guilt was quite obvious. Telling him that I had to go to the pharmacy to pick up the medication to begin the treatment for the infection, he promptly agreed to take me. The day before when I was tested he looked nervous as he wondered what I was planning to do after hearing the results of the tests. Strange enough I showed no emotion because I was dead inside. When he left for work that day it was late and I wondered if he had gone to commiserate with his woman after the day's event. I called his woman as soon as PaviElle went to take a nap because we had gone to the doctor very early and she was tired.

When the woman answered the phone I asked, "How could you have oral sex with a man you barely knew. A man you don't know if he is clean or contaminated? How could you sleep with a man while your teenage daughter is in the house? Are you not afraid of disease?" She did not answer my questions but began to give me all the details about her relationship with Lloyd from beginning to end, including the nights he slept at her house and took showers. She kept repeating he took showers, and gave vivid details of the wide variety of sex they had. She said she knew I would have called her again, and that she planned to tell me all she knew about my life so I would know she was not lying.

she knew everything. She expressed her disgust about the way he drank off her liquor, that he drank like a fish and were it not for the fact that he was wearing a wedding ring she would not have known he was married because I was not discussed. He only spoke about his daughter and what was happening to her. She again shared their sexual escapades and how much they enjoyed each other. I kept quiet and listened to every word while also taping the entire conversation. At the end of the call she told me I could call her anytime if I wanted to and she would be able to give me any information I needed. I told her thanks for the information but said there was no reason to call her again.

After the call, I tried my best to keep my rage in check. I rewound the tape to the beginning of the sordid conversation, and called Lloyd to listen to the voice of his mistress. He seemed to listen to the tape intently, not saying a word, but when the tape ended continued to lie and deny most of what she said, especially the part that he pursued her and called her several times to be with her. I then called his sister Sharon and his friend Blue and played the tape. They were speechless and shocked. I also went to my neighbor Roberta and played the tape for her. She was so hurt and felt so bad for me that she surprisingly proceeded to confess stories of her husband's infidelity hoping, I assumed, to give me some comfort on hearing her story. But, it did not work as nothing could comfort me.

When I heard Lloyd's car drive into the driveway, I ran outside and began to play the tape for him in person. He started to curse his woman and called her a liar, but he could not explain how she had everything else she said was a lie especially the part about him not being happy at home and needing to have someone to love him for who he was. I told him he must stop drinking and come clean and honest with his side of the story or I was leaving him and that he needed psychological help for what he had done to me and PaviElle. I told him he must also apologize to her because she was affected by his infidelity and disgusting behavior, and he agreed to do this. I then quoted the verse in the Bible about the fathers sins falling on the children and told him his sins were the reason why PaviElle got sick and was almost killed in the hospital. I was so filled with anger I wanted him to suffer and feel the betrayal and disgust I felt. I began hitting him to get him to talk and speak the truth, but the man stunned me by crying. I knew that night my firm opinion about not having guns in my house was absolutely right, because if I had one I probably would have shot my husband and possibly killed him.

The next day when I was taking PaviElle to therapy I realized that she was fully aware of what was going on with Lloyd when she said, "Mom, I heard Daddy crying last night."

She continued demonstrating what I was doing to him. I was surprised because she was fast asleep when I went to my bed. She said she woke up to use the bathroom and came close to the room to listen. She said she wanted to kill daddy. I told her no and we prayed for him and our family.

Later that afternoon Lloyd came home early and asked us to go with him to the mill shop to buy crown moldings. He got a call while we

Deadly Negligence

me if I was going to allow that woman to break up my marriage. June encouraged me, and said all we needed was counseling.

The next day after therapy I decided to drive to Coral Springs to let PaviElle visit my friend Joan, and called Judy to tell her about the tape. While we were at Joan's, Lloyd arrived home and kept calling me to find out where we were and who we were with. I did not answer the phone because I just wanted to get away and never see him again. When I finally decided to go home Simone called to ask how we were doing. We talked for a long time and then got PaviElle ready for bed. As usual Lloyd had fallen asleep in the chair and PaviElle decided to awaken him and tell him to take a shower and go to his bed. When he was in the shower I went into the bathroom and asked if that was the way he showered at his woman's house or if they did it together. He continued to lie, making denials as I watched him.

I put PaviElle to bed and then went to mine. When he came in the bed I told him I wanted more answers and needed him to tell me his version of the story, from the beginning because I knew their sordid affair began long before PaviElle got ill. As he began his side of the story, he asked if I remembered a woman who kept calling him numerous times stating that the job she hired him for was not done properly by one of his workmen, and she needed him to come to inspect the job.

As he spoke, I recalled the telephone calls and remembered him being disgusted. After inspecting the job he said she asked him if she could call him sometime and he said yes. Immediately I got irate and to injure my eye after hitting my head on the overhead cabinet I had begged him to remove. He had brushed it off and said I was getting old. I reminded him of the many times PaviElle had to tell him to leave me alone. I also reminded him of all the other incidents and told him to get counseling and I confessed that I did not know how to get pass what he had done to me. He said he had already apologized to PaviElle. I talked about his financial abuse that had forced me to have to sell Mary Kaye cosmetics, something I pledged never to do, to make ends meet. I finally felt he was starting to open up, but not totally.

I went to sleep but was awakened at 4:00 a.m. by PaviElle saying to me, "Please don't leave Mom." My reaction was one of confusion. What should my answer be I asked myself? I did not have an answer that was true so I hugged her, kissed her face and took her back to bed and promised to pray about her request. Although I failed to go back to sleep, I got up early so I could once again try to get Lloyd to confess. Maybe I was asking too much of him, or I was being sadistic, but I felt so desperate and at times my heart was beating so fast I thought I would explode and have a heart attack. Therefore I needed that confession to make me feel better.

Yes, I caught him early in the morning and I succeeded. He said I was right. He enjoyed the oral sex and that's why he kept going back and he did not use a condom, and he knew he had put both our lives in jeopardy. I told him he should call his sister Sharon, brother Wayne and cousin Yvonne to apologize for lying to them about it being a one night thing instead of a full blown relationship. I finally got my

Deadly Negligence

his former boss to get back his old job because he had too much time on his hands, owning his own business and that was the reason he found time to f... someone else.

After his confession I took refuge in my bathroom that night taking an endless shower like the one I took when I first got the bombshell news. I felt so dirty so I kept washing and washing as if I could wash it all off my inner and outer body. My overwhelmed state of mind remained daunting as I continued talking to myself and also asking God what I had done to deserve all this. First my daughter's near death, and now my husband's cheating. I thought of the sins of my father, a man I never met. Were they falling down on me? Or was it that some ridiculous witchcraft was the reason for all this suffering in my life?

My cousin saved me in my moment of grave weakness. She told me I should go back to my routine with my family and don't talk about the affair or say anything mean anymore. She reminded me of the Bible verse she gave me earlier, that said we have all fallen short of the glory of God and we all make mistakes. I tried very hard to take her advice but I just could not stop crying. I cried so much that Lloyd began to think I was getting a cold, and when he asked if I was sick my response was, "It is not a cold. I am crying because I want to know what I have done to you to deserve this?" Whenever I experienced symptoms of the infection he transmitted to my body, I would scream at and lash out at him. He started to believe in the effort I was making to take Marcia's suggestion to return to our family routine. He called me to say one of his women friend that he claimed he did not meet and he would have someone to talk with who would tell him the truth and he did. After his meeting with Sharon and we discussed her response and advice, I made a commitment to be in contentment, humility and gratitude, blessing everyone, including Lloyd who had so deeply punctured my heart and sense of trust. I also decided to resurrect my big dreams that I normally dream, and focus on restoring my daughter and my marriage. It was an extremely tough promise to keep and I had to later insist that we go to counseling with Prophetess Dr. Charmaine Peart.

Chapter 14

On Good Friday March 21 2008, at 5:00 a.m. I woke up, and then made PaviElle's bed because she had asked to sleep with us. As I made the bed there was a clear voice telling me to get my family up and go see the sunrise on Ocean Drive on the Island of Palm Beach. I did just that and it was the beginning of a long arduous, bumpy road filled with deep potholes and pitfalls, but a journey that was crucial to recapturing what we once had as a family filled with love. The trust would prove so much more difficult to rebuild after such betrayal. I believed in my heart and soul that my family needed a cleansing and a new beginning that seeing the sunrise and walking on the beach would be a good place to start.

We got there in time to see the spectacular sunrise and clear blue expansive ocean. We took lots of pictures and video as we braced the wind and sand, embracing each other in a group hug asking God to repair our family and give us back all that we had lost as he promised to do in his word - Joel chapter 2:25-27. 25 *And I will restore to you the years that the locust hath eaten, the cankerworm, and the caterpillar, and the palmerworm, my great army which I sent among you. 26 And ye shall eat in plenty, and be satisfied, and* pledged to make this a family tradition as long as we were in Florida on Good Fridays. We drove back home feeling healed and prepared to take on the difficult journey that we needed to save our family. When we got home I was thankful for a great morning, but though it was beautiful I personally was filled with mixed emotions; happiness, joy, sadness, sorrow and pain about what my husband, who I trusted and loved so much, had done. What a betrayal and deception I thought

Lloyd took us to work with him as if he wanted to hold on tightly to the feelings we had just shared at the beach and keep him out of trouble, or help to free his conscience. We spent the entire day together. The rocky road would continue when we discussed any of our friends who had committed the same sin as Lloyd. We would argue about small things and especially his idea that I should forget what he had done. I was just amazed at the way he was taking what he had done to PaviElle and I, asking questions like why it was so difficult for me to sleep at nights. I would snap and reply, "You don't seem to understand the magnitude of what you have done, and look at the Jeep that you hit twice saying nothing to me about it. I'm sure you hit it when you were visiting your woman." He would not respond which would only make me more lost, angry and overwhelmed.

We continued to do our routine family outings but there would always be something to trigger an argument. In the midst of all my marital turmoil I received a welcome call from Dr. Rubin. She said her friend Claudina, who had visited PaviElle in the hospital at Jackson Memorial, gave her a message to deliver to me. "She said to tell you had to be admitted to the hospital because of severe headaches. We prayed, and I told him not to worry because he would be fine.

Turning back to my marital problems, I asked Lloyd what he would do if I was the one who had cheated. He said he would not have called anyone, like I had done, and would consider it the "worse" aspect of our marriage vows and move on. I also asked if he was still the nice guy I thought I married, he said that he was. I explained to him that it was important to me to get the word of his infidelity out so in case I left him people would know it was not my fault and he should thank some of my friends like Joan who encouraged me to stay with him because her experience was much worse and she kept trying.

My cousin Marcia called almost every day and gave me scriptures to read, like Psalms 35, 37, 39, 40 and 91. She prayed with me constantly, begging and pleading with me to forget what had happened like she had done with her husband. On other days she asked me to say nothing more to Lloyd about the situation because he was ashamed and God would forgive him for what he did. She emphasized again that we all made mistakes and had fallen short of the glory of God and I should continue to be the wife of Proverbs 31–doing all the things I normally did to make my home a happy place, and loving Lloyd unconditionally. She emphasized that forgiveness was the real fulfillment of love, and reminded me that God forgave all His children although they sinned, and this was because God loved us unconditionally.

I kept saying that never happened to me until then. It did not seem fair to me that I would keep myself clean only to be contaminated by my husband's wanton appetite to satisfy his selfish needs during a time of such devastation in our family.

PaviElle kept improving and getting better at tasks like fastening the seatbelt in the car and calling her dad and me for group hugs. She was still getting frustrated with not being able to put on gloves, or not being able to wear her favorite open toe sandals because of her missing piece of toe and ugly scars. But, she would always recover quickly from her negative attitudes and smile again, but continued to express her displeasure with rehab. I had to constantly reassure her that she would see results in the future when she would be able to do normal things again.

An interesting event took place one night to put me back into attack mode with Lloyd. As I tried to wake him up to go take a shower, in his sleepy state he began babbling and I clearly heard him calling out his lovers name saying, "I am going home now" as if she was the one trying to awaken him. I wanted to kill him but went to my bed instead. When he came to bed later I confronted him with what he said but he did not believe me, which further enraged me. So to prevent a confrontation I plugged my ears with my head phones and listened to Yanni and Mozart until I fell asleep.

The next day I took PaviElle to the library. While she browsed through the books she liked, I looked at some design books and magazines to take my mind off my problems. I looked for a book my cousin went to another fabricator and got the job done correctly. I asked him to give me the telephone number for the woman and I called her. I told her that she should go ahead and call her lawyer and please let him know she had my husband's $750 and the granite we sent back, but I had nothing in return. I reminded her of the three day notice she failed to give Lloyd before she did the job, and told her I would report her to the Chamber of Commerce, Better Business Bureau, and I would also call some of the local TV stations to report her so they could feature her and her company in the programs they aired to warn consumers of being ripped off. I told her never to threaten my husband again with a law-suit, because while he may be a softie, I definitely was not. I told her that I would also report that she was charging customers twice the going rate of $30 per square foot for the product. Meekly, she responded, "Okay mam," and we never received another call from her or her imaginable attorney. This was a case of a another loss of money Lloyd had incurred, another mess which I had to clean up, while everyone was thinking I was a bitch and he was the nice guy.

The time came to visit Dr. Lue, the neurologist. He examined PaviElle and said her left hand was not spastic but had Dystonia. He said he wanted her to take another MRI and spinal tap and contact Dr. Lucy Cohen the physiatrist for a second opinion on the Botox injection. I wasn't feeling great about all his suggestions, but I complied and all the results from these new tests were good. However, I called Dr. Cohen. She said she had no guarantees about the Botox so once more I erased the thought.

not believe me. He tried very hard to be nice to me but it was not registering. He was so distracted that he left his tool pouch at the client's house and we had to return to Fort Lauderdale to pick it up

When we got back home after picking up PaviElle at Dr. Rubin, Marcia called before we went to bed and made what I thought was an outrageous suggestion. She said I should try to have sex with my husband after I took care of myself. I told her I was not ready for that at all. Lloyd heard me talking with her and asked what she had said, and I told him. He must have assumed I was prepared to heed Marcia's suggestion because when he came to bed he embraced me, and attempted to be amorous, but all I could think about was him being with his woman and all the things he might have told her, especially about our daughter and all the details of our personal life. Responding was tough, I thought, even as I tried to feel something. Early Saturday morning Lloyd was trying his best to cuddle and hug me. I felt his erection pressing against me, but my body could not respond as my mind was consumed with images of him and that woman. I returned his embrace but that was all I could give for the

It was the Sabbath Day and I had promised Prophetess we would visit her church to give a testimony of PaviElle's miracle healing. At first Lloyd said he could not go with us because he had a client, but I called him in the bedroom and told him my spirit was telling me he needed to be with us in church. He looked sad, but as usual had no response. By the time I walked to the laundry room singing, "God daughter, Ksandra, her son PJ and another relative, RJ. They gave her a beautiful rose and one of their song selections was, "I Sing Because I'm Happy." We had a great time and left after the offering was blessed so that Lloyd could make his appointment on time.

The following day we decided to clean house and we did it together as a family. It almost felt like old times. Lloyd went next door to help our neighbor Joey and they offered him a drink and he accepted, but I reminded him about his promise to me and I said no to the drink. I cried to Roberta and she encouraged me telling me that I must put what Lloyd had done behind me. She reminded me that she had gone through the same thing and was in the same position several times.

PaviElle expressed joy when she told me she saw Daddy kissing me. I could not explain to my daughter that I was trying hard but my body was not responding to her dad's efforts. Again, I was feeling unhappy, grateful and sad at the same time. The disappointment of Lloyd's cheating still consumed my thoughts but Prophetess called and averted my depression. She thanked us for visiting her church and sharing the testimony, and extended an invitation to go with her to North Carolina, New York and Baltimore to share the testimony. I told her about the website I had created and expressed my desire to raise funds for traveling and helping other families. She thought it was a great idea and promised to look at the website created for my daughter.

As PaviElle continued to make progress I got worried about her lip

Chapter 15

here was a significant and happy development on April 1, April Fool's Day, as it was also the first day of PaviElle's menstrual cycle which had returned in a normal fashion. The doctors and I were worried that because of the chemotherapy she may not have her period again. But God is an awesome God. Having her period back was very positive as long as she was at home and only going to therapy, but it created major challenges as soon as she returned to

The following day our happiness continued when I read the book, "The Secret." After reading the book, which I did in one night, I began to feel great. I made my husband and daughter watch the DVD of "The Secret" because it invigorated me so much. I began to tell myself that I will live my life in love, with great passion, and I knew more than before that I could have everything I wanted in life for me and my family. Later, when I started to analyze the book more deeply and I had a moment of revelation. I realized that most of the things stated in the book is in the Bible that I was constantly reading for comfort and hope. I was so filled with joy, and PaviElle showed such happiness after watching the DVD of "The Secret" she asked me to

Deadly Negligence

focused and her memory was being restored every single day. She became so addicted to her Nintendo DS that I began to wonder if I had made the right decision to purchase it. The advantages outweighed the negatives so I opted to make sure she did not play the games when she should be sleeping. She began to hide it under the sheet and instead of going to sleep she was busy playing the game. Every spare moment she had was devoted to the Nintendo DS.

Unfortunately, our state of peace, joy and marital repair would be interrupted by a call at 10:00 p.m. Luckily no one heard the telephone ring, but the woman Lloyd had the affair with had the gall to call that late in the night and leave a message on our voice mail. She wanted to know if he was okay. When he listened to the message he was furious and handed me the phone to listen to her message. We both talked about it and decided to go back to the rules of "The Secret." We had reorganized our den and living room so the chee could flow and remove the evil that had swirled around after the negative energy from the voice mail. We were not going to allow that woman the power to come into our home and derail our marital restoration. We hugged each other and he apologized over and over. My heart was beginning to heal and I began to feel a passion for my husband again because he had finally come clean and acknowledged my pain and disappointment in him.

In the early morning of April 4, Lloyd built up enough courage to caress me and massage my body. The time had come, and God in his glory allowed me to relax and we made love. I had accepted the fact in my heart and soul we had begun to heal as a couple and another

I was dumbfounded, not sure what to say or do in that moment. Quickly I gathered my thoughts, because I could see that Lloyd was crushed at what she was saying. I held her hands and explained that God forgives all our sins so it is the right thing for us to forgive each other also. Lloyd apologized to her again and we had an open conversation as a family, assuring her that it was fine for her to express herself and we wanted her to be happy. This incident must have affected her because the next morning at 6:00 she cried very deeply, saying, "I want to be back to my old self again."

We both had to tackle this by telling her she would be her old self soon but she had to be patient. We allowed her to cry for a very long time and talk about her feelings. I also encouraged her to read the book, "The Secret" because when she had watched the DVD she was very enthusiastic and hopeful about her recovery. After a while that felt like an eternity, and broke my heart, she stopped crying and surprisingly got up, got her waffles out of the freezer and fixed breakfast by herself. I asked her if making the waffles made her feel more like herself and she said, "Yes." On our way to therapy that morning I assumed we were successful in making her forgive Lloyd but I was wrong. She kept quiet, then burst out saying, "I am mad with Daddy because of what he has done."

I then asked her why she didn't say that to her father to his face when we had our family discussion, but she had no response. I shared the conversation with Lloyd when he got home and they both had another talk and she appeared to be better. He told her to sleep with us in our bed explaining that was a good way for all of us to get grader who made the principal's list was something she was happy to remember. In that environment students were taught songs to help them remember formulas and concepts in math and social studies.

She also became more self conscious about losing her hair, so I experimented with headbands and hats for a while, until her hair started growing rapidly again. She began remembering her friends like the Harts, and insisted we visit them the way we sometimes would in the past. Small things would make her upset during the process of her regaining her memory. For example when she found out visitors were occupying her bedroom at grandma's house, she kept calling her grandmother relentlessly and expressed such disapproval. This behavior caused me to be concerned because I thought about the doctors telling me that the brain injury may affect her personality. Lloyd on the other hand was making great effort to try and mend what was broken and be extra nice to us but some days he would revert to some mean action especially if he forgot to do something and we reminded him.

Our legal battles against the faulty hospital was heating up and Mr. Rosen brought his son Evon Rosen on board and introduced him to us by way of a conference call. Evon sounded compassionate and full of energy wanting mostly for our family to get the best possible compensation for the tragedy we experienced. He pleaded with me and convinced me not to direct my energy to anger because the damage had already been done to PaviElle, but rather redirect that energy towards getting maximum compensation. At first I thought my anger was well placed but realized that his advice and wise counsel

Evon joined the team Mr. Rosen said the hospital's attorney called to mediate the case before they filed the lawsuit. I was upset because I believed the hospital was trying to mediate quickly because to them my daughter was just another victim they needed to get rid of as quickly as possible.

My emotions were so raw and fragile that anything would set me into a crying frenzy. Lloyd got a little more sensitive to my feelings as our meetings with the Rosen's became more frequent and we had to do more depositions with the hospital's attorneys. I believed Mr. Rosen constantly congratulated him about being supportive and offered him stories about other men, who would have jumped ship and would have been unable to cope with the tragedy. After having found out about Lloyd's affair I felt sick to my stomach each time Mr. Rosen said this to him, but decided not to reveal his dirty little secret. I felt sick with hypocrisy but managed to inject this into my crying each time I had to rehash and tell what happened that awful morning of June 7, 2007. After each meeting I would tell Lloyd how I was feeling and he had no response but his guilt was apparent. He would try desperately to ramp up his show of affection until we got to a place where I would state how deeply I was affected and how hurt I felt because of his cheating but then he would apologize over and over. Our attempts to return to a normal sex life proved difficult but we still managed to make love sometimes when he was able to distract my visions of him with that woman and focus on our wonderful past experiences and memories.

PaviElle continued to have her struggles and victories, and it was had a great lunch together and Ursula decided to share her son and only child's story, with us. I was astonished to learn that her son was disabled from birth and had a learning disability but he would be graduating from college soon. Our hope meter flew through the roof as we listened to her son's struggles and triumphs, knowing that God had sent her to lift us up with her testimony. Dr. Rubin always had exceedingly great ratification and provided us with just the right prescription to continue the fight, no matter how difficult and steep climbing the mountain would become for PaviElle.

Chapter 16

new chapter began in our road to recovery on April 4 when I had to meet with the individuals at Okeeheelee Middle School who would make all the crucial decision about my daughter's return to school. The big reason for the meeting was to discuss what is called an IEP - Individual Education Plan. As I entered the room where the meeting was being held I felt like I was entering a pressure cooker, about to be tenderized without a choice. The room was filled with all the powerful decision makers from the School District of Palm Beach County and if I were a weakling I knew they would surely gobble me up. So, I quickly gathered myself and remembered that I was a television and radio talk show host who had anchored the evening news and created, produced and hosted the most successful television talk show in history in the Caribbean, and successful in London, England, and had interviewed prime ministers and celebrities, and was the youngest and first female director of news in Jamaica's history. So I said, "Wow, I think I should not have come alone but bring my own army." Everyone laughed and made great effort to put me at ease.

I knew in my mind that they would not overpower me and I would actually wanted to put PaviElle in ESE classes. I said absolutely not, remembering again that Dr. Jill Bolte Taylor, the author who had also suffered a brain injury, said always to return to what you did in your everyday life professionally or school and your recovery would be better and faster. Dr. Rubin reminded me of her friend Ursula and the intervention she had to do for her son. I left the meeting feeling embattled but thanked God for helping me through the tears and challenges.

Melissa also decided after testing PaviElle that it was time for her to do an audio program and PaviElle revealed to Malissa that she was remembering more about school. This was truly an awesome day for PaviElle who would visit her school on Wednesday after the meeting.

The occasion was organized by Grady, her homebound teacher, with our family all excited and in harmony with this event. She wore her new glasses and her friends took notice. They graciously complimented her short hair, her slimmer body and told her that her smile was just as beautiful as before. They welcomed her with open arms showing compassion for what she had experienced with the unfortunate tragedy but some seemed afraid of hugging her too tightly because to them she looked frail. Her special friends like Johnathan, Cloye and Lauren gave her a special card they had gotten which touched me so much, I cried.

All the students from her grade took turns to visit with her and took pictures. The teachers were not left out. These included, Dr. Rubin, Mr. Bender, language arts, Ms. Valdez, Spanish, Ms. Parrado, her. The visitors also included the school speech therapist and Ms. Barowski, the receptionist.

All the students were allowed to leave their classes to come and see PaviElle and assured her that when she returned to school they would make sure she got all the help she needed to succeed and return to the smart student she was, because while she was at school she was the one helping them with homework and other school work.

There were lots of hugs, kisses and stares with each person throwing questions as if we were at a press conference. It was an extremely gratifying and fulfilling day that would be cemented in my daughter's brain that showed that having good friends was an absolute blessing. She was shown so much love one would have to be present to soak up the atmosphere and witness those individuals in their most compassionate form. PaviElle had such a great time she wanted to stay at school instead of returning home. The trip was a success and her homebound teacher, Grady, was ecstatic and proud so she gave the approval for her to return to school the following week for short days, taking a few classes at a time until she felt ready to pursue a full schedule.

Ms. Santiago, her art teacher, did something that surprised everyone. She created a wood carving of PaviElle's name with incredible art work and beautiful bold colors and presented it to her at the event. The piece of art was gorgeous and it could be seen that Ms. Santiago had taken time to create something that PaviElle would cherish and appreciate for the rest of her life. What a fantastic welcome and a

Deadly Negligence

Our next stop was going to her best friend Jonathan's house. He had extended an invitation to visit his family. His mom and dad were very excited to see her, and his sister Sophie insisted on playing with her. Jonathan got PaviElle a beautiful bunch of flowers and we had a very long visit.

When we got home she was exhausted, so I made a good dinner. We were surprised that Lloyd was coming home early every day since his affair was exposed and he had promised to give up cheating. It was a good thing, but it kept me wondering how unbelievable and deceptive his behavior was. I knew all those evenings he came home late was not about work but about his woman for which he denied.Occasions like these made me revisit the memories of the sordid, unfaithful relationship he had, and kept lying about. I kept trying to figure out the exact time the affair started and calculated it to fourteen months. I did this by going back to the work schedule calendar and checked the months exactly to the day. It was definitely months before PaviElle got ill and experienced that awful tragedy.

After figuring out the timeline I asked him if he was with his woman the morning I called him about PaviElle almost being killed in the hospital. He said, "No, I was right here in the driveway packing up the truck to go to Fort Lauderdale to the job site." I was not convinced to this day, because he had taken a long time to come to the hospital after I had called him to deliver the devastating news.

It was now time to return to Atlanta to see Dr. Johnston, the physiatrist and all the other specialists that had worked with her in me and I kept unusually quiet because with so much time on my hand I kept thinking about Lloyd and his cheating. I just couldn't get it out of my head. I thought of the women I had watched on television over the years who said after they caught their husbands cheating and decided to stay to rebuild the marriage they became so consumed with the cheating itself they had to eventually leave. Was this going to be my fate also, or would I stay and become bitter and resentful, unable to erase it from my mind? I think I needed professional help but knew I could not afford the money it would cost as we needed every dollar to pay for all the things, extra therapies and tutoring PaviElle needed for her restoration. My needs were not that important. I vowed to take care of my problems and stop thinking about this affair. But this would prove more difficult than I anticipated. I was constantly asking God for his help.

Dr. Johnston was elated to see PaviElle and the tremendous progress she had made, and did a thorough examination. He recommended another treatment called Forced Use Therapy for her left hand that would take her to the next level. He wanted us to see the dentist, and pediatrician, Dr. Eppenbaum, who did a thorough physical examination including an ultra sound of her Thyroid and blood work. All was normal and my nerves were calmed, and I was thankful that God was truly working miracles.

April 21 was her second day to experiment with going to school for a short time and would leave when she got exhausted. When we arrived Ms. Parrado, her guidance counselor, met us outside and told us to enter the building after the crowd had gone inside so we sat

She was disappointed about not returning to school but we had to keep Dr. Lue's advice in mind and keep seizures from occurring. We continued to juggle short days at school and other days with Grady her Homebound teacher. This arrangement worked well for her and there were times when Ms. Santiago was doing something exciting in her class like connecting to the sister school in Spain on screen and PaviElle asked to stay. Going back to school full time had to be approved by Dr. Lue the neurologist. On April 23 she managed to write her first full paragraph about her day for Grady. She was also invited by the National Junior Honor Society (NJHS) students to help with career day because she was a member before her brain injury. She helped with career day and was taken care of by her friend Lauren who told me not to worry because PaviElle would be in good hands.

As we approached the end of April it was evident that Lloyd's business was slowing down as the economy headed into a recession. His former boss, Mr. Pomeroy, and owner of another company, had called and wanted him to come back to work for him. This was a welcomed idea by me, but Lloyd kept trying to hold out for a big contract he was working to land. I thought he was being stubborn and not seeing what was happening with the economy, but I decided to say nothing more in fear of getting my feelings hurt with his harsh answer. I pledged never to bring up the subject again. Finally, one day he called me to say that he had spoken to Mr. Pomeroy and he had an appointment to meet with him the following day. He asked us to go with him and we did. The day was positive and he was offered his old job back. I was somewhat cynical as I asked him if he would like me to tell Mr. Pomeroy about his cheating on me because he was work because there were secrets and distrust and most of all I no longer felt any love for him. He snapped and said, "We will work." I tried to make him understand that I was trying and every day I asked God to help me, but I was unable to feel any passion or love for him. There were so many incidents, large and small, that would trigger my memory and make me remember the affair. All he had to do was raise his voice while speaking to me, or answer my questions or comments in a way that I thought was uncaring and I would snap reminding him of the pain and suffering he had caused our family.

PaviElle made a request that she wanted to take a walk around the complex where we lived, something we always did as a family every week. We were caught off guard because in the past when we walked she complained, and was happy when it ended. We took the walk and she never complained but she was upset that she was not yet able to ride her bike. I congratulated her for her strength during the walk and told her one day she would be capable of riding her bicycle

Life can be unusual sometimes, because the person who comforts you in your time of distress may need your shoulders to cry on later. This became so clear to me one morning at 6:35 a.m. when my home phone rang and I wondered who could be calling so early, especially on the house phone. I jumped out of bed as quickly as I could to avoid waking up the entire household. To my surprise the sobbing voice on the other end of the line was my cousin Marcia who had provided me so much comfort during the pain I endured in the days and weeks after I learned of Lloyd's cheating. She was crying

My struggles were constant, but on the days that Prophetess called the burden felt lighter and thought filled. She said there had to be something she could do to lighten my burden and give me a break. She offered to get a crew to clean my house and have her husband Peter, who is a great cook, come to my house and cook for our family. At first I resisted, but she insisted. I shared with her my feeling of despair and she counseled me saying God had chosen me because I was special and He never gives us more than we can bear. I told her, I felt that I had gotten more than my share. At the time I was tempted to tell her that Lloyd had cheated on me but I could not find the words. The journey seemed like there was no end in sight. The cleaning did not take place, but the dinner was fantastic and the nicest thing anyone had done for our family for a long time. We had a great time and the gesture was appreciated by everyone.

Again I wondered what had happened to all my friends who used to call me almost every day to talk about their problems. Friends like Betty and Sandra Lee, Barbara, and to a lesser degree, Joan and Judy. I later found that they were afraid to call and not knowing what to say. I thought that was not a valid excuse, because if any of my friends had problems I was always there in person or calling all the time. So what was different when I had the problem? Sandra Lee said she just could not bring herself to see PaviElle in her current brain injured state and Joan said sometimes she wanted to call but just did not know what to say. All I wanted was for them to call and ask how I was doing and let me know they were thinking of us. At one point I decided to start calling everyone and give them an update as to how her recovery was going, but a light bulb went off in my head and one daughter Monique, were nurses and there was nothing that would come up that they could not handle. She just wanted me to take a break. PaviElle no doubt had a wonderful time and fell in love with Monique who she said was so nice to her although she was meeting her for the first time.

I learned reluctantly that life is not about what you would do for your friends in their tragic times, but which of your friends would step up and be there for you in your own tragedies. This is the reality of life. Friends do not necessarily stay around when you are down, no matter how close you think you are.

Joan, my best friend who is also PaviElle's god mother, made excuses for herself most of the times and she certainly tried sometimes, but I believe seeing my daughter reminded her of her own tragedy when her only child, Joey, died within hours at a hospital. We are still convinced his demise came by way of negligence the way my child also experienced devastation. I felt blessed, Joan once told me that although PaviElle suffered a brain injury and would have disabilities she was alive, but Joseph was dead with no chance of recovery. I repeated her words to myself frequently when I begin to feel depressed and it continued to provide me with an instant reminder of the miracles God sent me. In writing this book I feel like I am also doing it for Joey.

Chapter 17

Returning to school as a full time student caused PaviElle some anxiety as she told me, "Mom I am nervous about school." Meanwhile the legal battle was moving fast. The attorneys, ours and the hospital's, had ramped up their demands from us, including various test that PaviElle was required to take to satisfy them. Her first big test was with Dr. Foreman, involving a long initial telephone interview with me. This was followed by a home visit and interview with all of us and then with our permission, PaviElle alone. The interview was extremely long, emotional and exhausting but was necessary for Dr. Foreman to create a Life Plan for PaviElle now and in the foreseeable future. He was thorough and left nothing out of his extensive report. There were items he listed to help PaviElle which we never knew existed and his life plan was called the Rolls Royce Plan which had to be changed and adjusted several times based on the prosecution's request.

The interview with Dr. Foreman was extremely difficult and emotional for me. I cried the entire time not only because I had to relive the tragedy from the beginning, but also because he asked Lloyd and I how was our marriage as he wanted to recommend counseling. Lloyd felt the need to lie because in his mind that was the result he was truly hoping for our marriage. I allowed it to pass and tried desperately to regain what was lost in my heart and soul but the pain and mind games continued to torment me every day. All the therapists had to engage in their own tests which was extra work for them. This really became overwhelming and unnecessary at times but had to be done. The speech pathologist, Malissa, had to do hearing and audiology testing that was exhausting for my daughter. There were many more, including one by the school psychologist, Joanne. Her test was not enough for the hospital's attorneys so we had to travel almost two hours to Miami for three days to do another psychological test with Dr. Hamilton after she returned to school full time.

I grasped very quickly that in a legal battle, even though the evidence was so clearly in your favor, there still would be several mountains to climb, holes to sink in, and possible drown in the sea of paperwork that are destined to kill numerous trees. The repetition of the same tests multiple times was my biggest frustration. It appeared to me that the hospital attorneys were constantly requesting the same forms and paperwork to show their client they were earning their fees. The legal system in America is one we had no desire to tangle with but had no choice, and I for one learned legal terminologies very fast, what it entails to sue a hospital for malpractice and, what I kept pointing to as obvious negligence. I had to take PaviElle to one expert or specialist after another always with the same conclusion. I had taken my normal only child to the hospital and because of the refusal to listen to my adamant insistence about her not getting Versed, they gave it to her anyway. The devastating consequence

All the therapies and tutoring given through the school district continued until PaviElle returned to school full time. The speech therapist Ernestine, the only African American therapist we encountered in Florida, made us a miraculous offer that was God's favor. She said she would continue to see PaviElle for speech until she was doing better and when I asked her how much it would cost me she said, "Nothing." I thanked her over and over because she was very good with PaviElle and gave me a great deal of information that I needed to know to make sure she received all the benefits that was offered by the system for disabled children.

When she finally left us because of other pressing commitments I was very sad but she assured us that she would only be a telephone call away if we needed her. The extra time she invested with PaviElle was very helpful and helped her tremendously.

We needed to take one more trip to Atlanta for the summer which would also include the meeting with Raven Simone at Six Flags. We were picked up by a stretch limousine but when we arrived at the park they had no passes for us and no one knew what we were talking about.

I called Raven's representative and the problem was finally resolved. I was not very impressed with the preparation. I tried my best to be civil to Lloyd so as not to spoil the day for PaviElle because on our way to Atlanta he said something and I responded with the words of his woman, "You are the one who is not happy at home and wanted to be loved for who you are."

because Raven did not even have a conversation with her and the camera they provided was defective. We took a cell phone picture when Raven signed the picture that they eventually took. They finally invited PaviElle on stage and she had a good time but for me the event fell short of our expectation. But, my daughter was happy and that was most important.

The situation with Lloyd and I percolated into another day. He left the house to get juice for PaviElle by himself although I was dressed and wanting to go with him so we could be alone and have a conversation about the anger I was feeling towards him. When he returned I asked why he left me and he apologized saying all the other days he was going alone so he did not know I wanted to go with him. I reminded him that this was the way he behaved before I found out about his woman and opted to go wash my mother's car alone so he could call his woman and keep her up to date about what he was doing. I asked him what were his plans because I would not put up with his cheating again. He apologized and said, "I may be stupid but not a fool." My mom had a good laugh at his remark and we went about

Later we went to Brazelton, Georgia in search of products for my Aunt Lucille, but a strange thing happened when PaviElle, Mom, Lloyd and I were in the car. She pushed her dad in the back of his head and said, "You are too sex crazy."

Mom and I froze with our mouths wide open and I almost stopped breathing as the atmosphere became tense and extremely

Deadly Negligence

My mother joined in and counseled her granddaughter who she realized was hurting quietly because of what Lloyd had done. I actually felt embarrassed for my husband, but there was nothing I could have said to him that would change the way his daughter was feeling. As we entered the store he hugged her and spent most of the shopping trip talking with her and reassuring her that he was sorry for what he had done. By the time we left, tension was lifted and things appeared normal for the moment. On our way back from Atlanta my mind was jumping and I blurted out to Lloyd, "Are you worried that your woman could be pregnant?" He replied, "I am not worried about anything."

Chapter 18

he summer of 2008 was fast approaching its end. PaviElle and I picked up the supply list for school and she was super excited as we went to WalMart to pick up her supplies. It was so pleasing to see her as she went through the isles to pick out the items. It almost felt like old times, but a strong reminder that she had missed one year of school and the road ahead would be filled with challenges and victories. I had to finalize all the arrangements for her return to Okeeheelee Middle School on a full time basis.

The process got very frustrating and combative with different people at the School Board led by Amy in charge of the IEP, and Laurie who was in charge of the Home Bound School Program, who convinced Dr. Lue the neurologist, that PaviElle needed to go back to school, integrate the district therapists and get approval for a one on one caretaker for her during school hours. I made an executive decision to call Dr. Samore, the principal of Okeeheelee to enlist his help in clearing up all the confusion and misinformation. As predicted, he called me back and gave me all the pertinent decision making individuals and their numbers at the school district to call.

I quickly got the wheels turning and all the road blocks were cleared

PaviElle would have to like the individual and there were certain things the aide was not paid to do like cleaning her up when she used the bathroom. I fought that hitch and got the school board members in charge of this to agree to pay for all the assistance necessary for my daughter's safety.

August 18, 2008 was the first day of school and we were blessed with a gorgeous sun filled, brilliant blue sky morning. PaviElle was filled with joy and was awake at 6:00 a.m. She got dressed with my help and we went to therapy at APS before making our way to school. All the therapists told her how great she looked and did everything to boost her confidence and self esteem before she faced her friends and teachers.

When we got to Okeeheelee the traffic was horrific so I had to change my route and use the front gate, which I was allowed to use because of her handicap tag. I kept in mind the advice given to me by Ms. Parrado when we went for the school visit and waited outside until all the other students had entered the building. We sat in the car for a while and I was the only one nervous as she was filled with excitement to go to class and feel normal again.

The confusion continued because of the method used by the school for students to find their home rooms. Eventually we were rescued by Ms. Valdez, who led us to the epicenter of chaos to the right information. Mr. Bender's room was the correct home room but PaviElle's name was not on the list. I had to find Ms. Parrado the guidance counselor who eventually sorted out the confusion after and present, and what her needs would be. I filled him in and then went to meet with Ms. Kelley in the eighth grade office but found Ms. Wood, the new ESE coordinator, who had a chip on her shoulder from the start. She invited me into her office and appeared to be helpful; promising to take all of PaviElle's needs into consideration and make sure she would have everything she was entitled to. Predictably, she turned out to be the enemy and an obstructionist.

With the decision made that I could stay with her at school until Dr. Samore hired a suitable aide, I was given a spot in Dr. Rubin's office, where PaviElle would be able to eat her lunch daily. The first day experience at the cafeteria was a disaster because the food was horrible, totally disgusting and repulsive but it was raining so hard I could not go out to buy her lunch. It was clear to me then why she always complained about the lunch at school and did not eat most of the time. I apologized to her and promised to fix her lunch every day going forward. At the end of her first full day of school her confidence sky rocketed so I stood back and allowed her to navigate her way through the crowded hallway when the bell rang.

She showed her responsible side and waited for me when the mass of students crowded the exit door. I was very proud to observe her strength and determination to be independent especially because she had declared that she did not need an aide to babysit her, all she wanted was for me to be there to take her to the bathroom. I was quite content to be at her service, something I had become accustomed to doing.

Deadly Negligence

professional volunteer at the school during her time in class and my service was appreciated by the staff.

On our way home from school on that first day, PaviElle began to cry. As I watched the tears rolling down her face and how sad she looked my heart sank because I knew her expectations of her friends reaction to her was not realized. She tried hard to hide her feelings but I kept asking what was wrong and showed my concern. When we got home I enlisted the help of my neighbor Roberta to talk with her. We both explained to her that missing her friends in Atlanta was okay, but she needed to keep in mind that they did not call to find out how she was doing or showed any concern about her well being. She was sad that Renee did not call and her friends at Okeeheelee seemed distant. I counseled her and eventually she heard me and accepted what I was telling her. She got all her yearbooks and looked through them thoroughly and felt much better.

With the approach of Hurricane Fay to South Florida, there was continuous heavy rain so school was cancelled the next day. Then the following day she did not want to go back to school so I had to encourage her and assure her that I would be there in case she wanted to leave. However, her anxieties disappeared and she had a great and better day. She began to demonstrate to me the things she remembered, like playing dress up and modeling by doing the model walk I had taught her. She remembered Owen and the name of the car dealership where we had purchased our Jeep. I knew her memory was being restored and I was filled with joy and thankful to God for his blessings.

walk close to her in the hallways for her safety and was very resistant to the idea of being assigned an aide. If I was not continuously occupied at the school, my tears would come falling down my cheeks without any effort, as my thoughts of her struggles at school with reading comprehension, writing, math, science, history and Spanish was evident. She was being seen as this fragile person that could no longer excel the way she did in the past. I so resented that as I knew she only needed time to restore her memory and intelligence. All the therapists were convinced that going back to school was helping her progress and she was a trooper about the entire journey.

The first week at school was a success, but we were both exhausted. She sensed my being tired and when I was washing her hair she said, "Mom, you can't be tired of me because it was you who gave me breath." I laughed and assured her that I would always be there for her and promised she would be good again.

She took her first test in Mr. Bender's class related to the book 'Mango Street' and scored 21 out of 30. Her disappointment was obvious but I assured her that she did great and every test would be better.

Another big meeting was scheduled with the IEP team. There were thirteen people from the school district and all of PaviElle's teachers. The meeting was long and intense at times. I cried when Mr. Bender stood to give his report and observations about PaviElle's return to school. He praised her for the test she took in his class and the good story she wrote and stated he was so impressed with her efforts and progress. Ms. Mansour her math teacher who was

Deadly Negligence

District Director that PaviElle would get an aide and all adjustments must be made for her to be successful in school.

At the meeting I fought hard for my child and made it clear that I was upset with the County for trying to put her in 9th grade when I had made it clear at the previous IEP meeting that she needed to do 8th grade work at Okeeheelee because of the brain injury and memory loss. This I said would be beneficial for her because she would be among a familiar support system of teachers, counselors and some friends. At that point we realized that the County had placed PaviElle in high school at Palm Beach Central and that was the reason her name was not in the computer or on the list at Okeeheelee. "What craziness," I thought, "Why did we have the first IEP meeting? Was no one listening to me?" The school system was simply flawed and incompetent, I concluded.

Dr. Samore, principal, Joanne Byron, school psychologist and Ms. Parrado, guidance counselor, all agreed with my decision and backed my argument for wanting that to happen. The most ridiculous decision made at the meeting was to make PaviElle take the FCAT examination. I was adamant that in her current state she would not be able to complete such a comprehensive exam after being out of school for one year recovering from a tragic brain injury and disability. The crew from the District said if she did not take the FCAT she would not get a regular high school diploma, but rather some alternative certificate. I decided to go along with the decision because in my heart I knew that PaviElle would not stay in the public school system for high school. I would do all the research that was necessary to find

After waiting for several weeks and there was no aide hired to assist my daughter I decided to discuss the matter with Ernestine, the speech therapist, and asked for her help. She promised to discuss the problem with Ms. Eversano. The following week she got back to me saying that Ms. Eversano was surprised that the aide had not started working with PaviElle as yet and I was still at the school with her all day. I told her that my information was that an aide was hired but was being vetted by the district. Ernestine relayed my concern and I continued to wait.

The entire back-to-school experience was filled with insanity, inconsistences, conflict and especially dealing with the crazy Ms. Dow who seem to hate the fact that children with disabilities and parents are not entitled to the benefits they receive. She tried to block or hinder every decision that was made at the IEP meetings.

After June Eversano had made all the decisions about addressing my daughter's needs at the IEP meeting Ms. Dow came to Dr. Rubin's office to inform me that the district had a hiring freeze and they could not hire an aide for PaviElle, but the district sent a substitute teacher. She added that the substitute teacher would only help my daughter with physical things like bathroom and carrying her back pack. I told Ms. Dow that was not what was discussed in the IEP meeting with Ms. Eversano. I followed her to her office and she was quite curt and rude but I persisted and she basically asked me to leave her office. She gave me the telephone number for Ms. Eversano, but told me I could not make the call in her office. I tried the number and it was incorrect. When I told her this, she got more irate and said, "I took me into her office after observing how frustrated I was with Ms. Dow and that I was crying. She called Ms. Eversano and then emailed her to explain what Ms. Dow had told me and why the aide was not yet serving PaviElle. I later saw Dr. Samore and told him what Ms. Dow told me about the hiring freeze. He said he was in the same IEP meeting with June Eversano where the decisions were made and they were aware of the problems with Ms. Dow and it would be taken care of. He put his arms around me and tried to reassure me that it would be okay.

After all the drama and misinformation from Ms. Dow, Ms. Rusch and I went to PaviElle's math class where the substitute teacher was and asked her what instructions were given to her by the district for PaviElle's care and needs for academics. She said they told her to do, "Anything she needs." We discussed all the subjects she would help PaviElle with and she said she was good at all subjects except Spanish. I told her thanks and went back to my position in Dr. Rubin's office. I could not believe Ms. Dow blatantly lied about the situation. I was now convinced that she was secretly crazy and should not be working with parents and students who were emotionally fragile who needed to work with someone who is compassionate. She further lied to the substitute by telling her she should wait for PaviElle in the 8th grade office in the mornings instead of the front door. I addressed the issue and the aide called out Ms. Dow when she tried to deny what she had told her. I took my copy of the IEP minutes to Ms. Rusch and showed her where it clearly stated that the aide who would be hired will help PaviElle with academics and all her bathroom needs. Ms. Parrado, the guidance counselor came and told me not to worry but asked how much more I could take. I was immediately reminded by my inner voice that disasters in one's life came in threes and my mom's accident was number three following PaviElle's brain injury and Lloyd's affair. I felt physically, mentally and emotionally drained, but I dug deep within me and told myself quitting was not an option. My mother's call was soon followed by the insurance company to say that the truck driver was suing for injuries. I went off on the phone telling the lady the sequence of the story my mom had told me. I asked her how the driver who was in a big truck could be claiming injuries, when his truck was hit in the rear by a Mercedes Benz SUV when he stopped suddenly. That was criminal, I said, and she assured me they would have a thorough investigation.

My mom was totally shaken by the accident and no longer wanted to drive. I did my best to encourage her and rebuild her confidence. After going to court and paying the undeserved ticket I convinced her to buy another car six months later. There was some help for me when Malissa, the speech pathologist, told me that she needed to speak with all of PaviElle's teachers and tutors to explain the method of teaching that would be most effective for her. She explained that with history, she needed large images in color for maps and anything involving graphics. For math and science, they must teach her pictorially and with repetition. Our Saturday sessions of tutoring with Dr. Rubin came to an end because she wanted to use the time to work on writing her math book. She would see PaviElle after school to continue the tutoring. Ms. Valdez also volunteered to tutor her in Spanish, Ms. Stover, language arts, and Mr. Thomas with science. I was extremely grateful for their help. It meant longer days for

Deadly Negligence

defeated and God was totally in charge.

The day finally came for the first aide to start working with PaviElle after I had sorted out all the other issues. When I took PaviElle to school there was no one there to meet us so I went to the front office to speak with the receptionist, Ms. Barowski. She had no answers for me but tried her best to help. I then went to Dr. Samore's office and spoke to his secretary, Ms. Ecirp, who was very curt, abrupt and unfriendly with me. She directed me to Ms. Dow, the enemy. Ms. Barowski seeing my distress offered to radio Ms. Dow who replied saying, "I am sitting in a class for Ms. Campbell and cannot deal with it now."

I could not believe what was happening. I felt like there was a secret conspiracy to make my life miserable and stop my daughter from receiving her benefits. Incredibly, the aide had been sitting right there in the office and said nothing. When I asked why she had remained silent among the confusion, she simply said she did not want to say anything. I thought to myself, "This crap is totally unbelievable." But, I ignored the silliness and introduced myself to her. She told me her name was Barbara and explained her experience working with students with brain injuries and told me about her good rapport with a young man who was in her care prior to the new appointment to take care of PaviElle. Cognizant of all the confusion about her appointment, and the incident in not locating her earlier, I told her no one really cares, to which she responded that she did care.

Later on Ms. Dow walked into the office with her head held straight went ahead to Ms. Block's room and they followed. Ms. Dow again was very rude as she spoke to PaviElle and introduced Barbara to them without including me and ignored my presence. After she continued to ignore me I asked Ms. Dow if I had a say in the matter and Ms. Block sensing the disrespect I was getting, and how upset I was jumped in and said, "Sure." I listened as everyone explained the routine PaviElle had with Runanda, the substitute teacher, and all her needs.

After it was all sorted out I wanted to tell Ms. Dow how I felt but instead I went back to Dr. Rubin's office and sobbed. She tried to comfort me and I then called Ms. Barowski to thank her for caring and trying to help. She said she was happy to help and understands my frustration.

I kept asking myself how the district could have hired someone like Ms. Dow who was so abrasive and uncaring with such an unfriendly personality. The good news was Barbara connected with PaviElle, but then she was dismissed after a short time because of her poor attendance record. I tried to plead her case, trying to prevent my child from being exposed to several individuals but this would prove to be a torching experience for me and my child. They pointed to the fact that Barbara was on her cell phone too much in class when she should be taking notes for PaviElle. This had caused PaviElle to wet her pants because she allowed her to pull her button by herself and she did not do it fast enough. Then there was the incident when I was called to bring a change of pants immediately because Barbara could not be found and PaviElle was seeing her period, went to the

Deadly Negligence

use the phone and she was sorry. I kept my cool but the information had travelled to quite a few people including those at the district. I got PaviElle cleaned up and rushed back to Mr. Bender's class, I kissed her assuring her that I was not mad and what happened was not her fault. Ms. Dow was also upset that Barbara was eating lunch with PaviElle in Dr. Rubin's office and told her she had to eat her lunch in the cafeteria only but I could stay with PaviElle in the office to have her lunch.

These things to me appeared to be small stuff in light of all the important needs facing my child. Barbara being Jewish had left early because of the Jewish holiday and this also became an issue that prevented me from fighting for her to stay as PaviElle's aide. She had also forgotten PaviElle one morning at the front door and she did not find her until 10:30 a.m. after a student told her where my child was. Barbara explained to me what happened and all was well.

Another issue rose again with Barbara, Amy Nworb and Ms. Dow about how much bathroom assistance PaviElle would need so she can get paid accordingly. I pointed out to them that when my daughter was seeing her period there was a serious problem with her changing herself. They said they did not remember to take that into consideration. I was totally annoyed at this point and wondered if my child was the first child they dealt with, that had a brain injury or disability. Was it necessary for me to point out in detail what exactly was included in bathroom assistance? I thought simple common sense would prevail. Amy Nworb responded saying she thought, PaviElle only needed help with opening and closing her pants according to that PaviElle would have to take. I only found out about the exam because Ms. Stover saw us in the lobby looking distraught because we were just fluffed off by Mr. Rivas the Spanish teacher who asked if she was prepared and volunteered to help her. When I asked Barbara about the exam she said there was nothing to study for. I explained to her that PaviElle is not a regular student and needed to be prepared for all exams in advance. She said sorry for the error and it would not happen again. I told myself that Ms. Stover was an angel sent by God through his son Jesus, as I expressed my gratitude.

When Barbara was informed that she was being removed and placed at another school, she called the district and was told that I did not like her and no longer wanted her to be PaviElle's aide. I was shocked and told her I had no such conversation with anyone.

I asked Dr. Samore and he said that could be his fault because the information came from him but by the time it was filtered through the district his words might have been distorted. He apologized for putting me in an awkward position with Barbara but said PaviElle needed someone that would be more reliable and dependable.

Although there was all this confusion PaviElle told me she was beginning to make new friends and was feeling very happy. My heart was filled with joy and thanking God that through the storm there was a ray of sunshine to save my soul.

A new aide, Ms. Etienne, was assigned to PaviElle after Barbara was transferred, and thankfully she was bilingual. Ms. Dow introduced her to us and all PaviElle's needs were explained in detail and I to the bathroom since he could not obviously assist her as he was a man, he responded, "I guess by herself." I left him and immediately went to Dr. Samore's office and told him I needed his ears urgently, demanding that he investigate the matter and call Ms. Dow to his office for an urgent meeting. I explained the male aide, and all other issues and road blocks I was experiencing with Ms. Dow. He listened keenly and took out his copy of PaviElle's IEP report and quickly flipped through the pages. When Ms. Dow arrived I was already crying hysterically, asking how could they have a man taking care of my 14 year old brain injured daughter on a one-on-one basis. What would happen when she needed to use the bathroom, I asked, and would they both like that to happen to their teenage daughter. Ms. Dow said she told PaviElle she should come to her office and get her if she needed to use the bathroom. I told Ms. Dow that was ridiculous because when PaviElle needed to use the bathroom, she would pee in her pants by the time she had to get her in her office then go to the bathroom. I used as an example, the incident that occurred with PaviElle when she peed in her pants, because Barbara was on her cell phone and not pulling her pants fast enough. Dr. Samore told Ms. Dow to solve the problems immediately and sort it all out.

I went back to Dr. Rubin's office and wept. I felt so overwhelmed and kept asking God what have I done to deserve all this. PaviElle had never hurt anyone so why was she suffering that way. I called a friend and told her what had happened, she told me I could sue the district for what happened. I did not pursue the thought because there was another lawsuit against the hospital and the intensive care doctor who almost killed my daughter.

PaviElle because she needed the social interaction with her peers. I called Lloyd and told him all that took place and he was also mad. He asked me not to worry. I also spoke to all the teachers who said they were not informed about the scheduling of the exams but assured me it would not happen again. I also called Ms. Rusch and made her aware of the mistake made having PaviElle take all exams in one day and not following the IEP. Ms. Dow's main concern was sending a questionnaire to all of PaviElle's teachers for her progress.

This was an extremely stressful time, but I told Joanne Byron the school psychologist God would see me through this difficult time. She saw me and asked how things were going and I could not stop to talk with her because my eyes were filled with tears as my voice cracked when I tried to answer her. I think she knew I was crying so she told me things would get better. Ms. Dow did not inform the teachers about giving my child a copy of each textbook to keep at home but tried to convince Dr. Samore that if she knew PaviElle needed help with opening and closing her pants she would have recommended as an alternative, elastic waist pants. I shot that idea down instantly, stating that I do not want my child to feel different and excluded. The mantra was "inclusion" for students with disabilities to prevent them from being isolated. The next day Ms. Etienne would surface again as the new aide.

Lloyd began stepping up his help with math and I did science, history, Spanish, language arts and art. Sometimes PaviElle felt overwhelmed and we had to slow down until she was ready to go again. Her determination got stronger each day so we had to work

PaviElle. I had to be the aide because Ms. Etienne wasn't there and one Ms. Kelley shows up with two other children and said she was also told to take care of my daughter. I asked her how could she manage to take care of three disabled children at the same time. PaviElle reacted with disgust and I told her, "Don't worry my sweet girl; mom is your aide for the day. And she replied, "Good."

I again complained to Dr. Samore about the situation and he was in disbelief about the same problem resurfacing all the time. Later on that morning Ms. Etienne arrived and took responsibility for her again. This was crazy I told Ms. Etienne. This day's uncertainty took a toll on both PaviElle and myself unexpectedly. We both had a major melt down and cried and cried then told Lloyd exactly how we felt about everything including his disappointing affair. It is quite strange how we try so hard to forget the bad things that happen in our lives but something happens that triggers all the bad feelings and pain.

In a matter of days, unbelievably, the aide problem returned. It was lunch time and Ms. Etienne came to inform us that another aide would take over immediately. This time her name was Amanda. Both PaviElle and I were so annoyed we had no response. However, I refused to erase the joy I was feeling about the possibility of a new President, Barack Obama.

This was one of the days I had indicated I would volunteer for his election campaign and I would not allow any other event to steal my joy. My days of volunteering for the Obama campaign were filled with optimism and I knew his victory would show my daughter that all was met by other supporters it became a festive affair. When I held up the signs reminding drivers to vote they would hunk their horns with hands waving with visible jubilation. History was about to be made in the great United States of America.

As the time drew near to pick PaviElle up from school I found myself so filled with excitement I could barely pull myself from the sidewalk to return the sign. I kept the sign and took it with me later that evening to the Crowne Plaza Hotel for the victory celebration. After I picked up my daughter from school I took her to the election offices where I was volunteering so she could get a feel for the hard work and dedication ordinary people like myself were doing for the Obama campaign. This was the perfect moment for us to forget our tragedy and enjoy the eminent history that was about to be made in our great country. My daughter got excited and later encouraged me to go to the celebration at the hotel. I called Winsome, a lady I had met at the election office and asked if she would accompany me to the hotel and she said yes. As we arrived at the hotel we struggled to find a parking space but could hear the noise and feel the energy coming from the ballroom. With my sign in hand we entered the packed room. People were everywhere. I found a great spot and held up my sign very high and jumped up each time Obama won a state.

I was standing beside Palm Beach Mayor Frankel the entire time and spoke to her but was so filled with glee I forgot to introduce myself to the mayor. I cried with tears of joy as I watched all the different people, whites and blacks, at the event hugging each other with nothing but happiness for being a part of a great historic moment in exchanged friendly conversation with me, had taken my picture with the sign and the picture appeared on the front page of the Palm Beach Post the next day in the newspaper's pictorial feature of the event. Lots of people I knew kept calling to check if it was really me even though the photographer had listed my name.

The experience of Obama's victory and the event I attended was exhilarating and recalled my pleasant memories of working for President Jimmy Carter's campaign. I knew that people were expecting way too much from the new president but trusted that God was in charge and would guide our nation through with a great deal of endurance and patience.

The morning after the election as I drove PaviElle to school I used President Obama's victory to affirm that she could be anything she wanted to be with hard work and determination while trusting God.

Getting to school put a damper on both our spirits because there was no aide again and when I enquired I learned Ms. Dow would be the aide until the district sent yet another substitute teacher to assist my child. As someone who truly believes there are no impossibilities with God I talked to myself, saying thanks to President Barack Obama for giving me one day of total joy after almost two years of sadness, disbelief and frustration about what had happened to my normal child when I took her to the emergency room on May 29, 2007, and they damaged her brain on June 7 2007.

When the time for another IEP meeting arrived, Ms. Dow again that day, but no one knew the answer. I asked how would they feel if their 14 year old daughter was assigned TEN different individuals on different occasions to be taken to the bathroom. I shouted that this was unacceptable, and then had another major meltdown.

The school psychologist was in her office and came out saying she heard my distress and invited me into her office. I totally lost it, and Ms. Rusch came running in with Ms. Rushenbaum and then Dr. Samore. With all of them in the very small office I again asked how would they feel if their 14 year old daughter was exposed to ten different people taking her to the bathroom. They all had stunned looks on their faces and were most likely thinking I was having a nervous breakdown caused by the school and the district. They all expressed they felt my pain and disappointment, but I told them I would be calling my attorney Evon Rosen to seek a solution. I emptied out my soul about the treatment and disrespect I was given and shown by Ms. Dow and her refusal to follow the IEP minutes. I told Dr. Samore that Ms. Dow behaved in a way that made me feel she did not want my child to receive the services she was entitled to. I said it was obvious that she hated me and PaviElle based on the way my daughter told me she treated her when I was not around. Clearly, I said, something was very wrong with this picture. Ms. Rusch left the meeting to see who was taking care of PaviElle before the bell rang and Joanne said she felt my pain so much she began to cry with me, hugged me and said, "I'm sorry." Dr. Samore asked me to tell him all the things that PaviElle was not receiving that were in the IEP and I did a thorough run through. He then ordered Ms. Dow to schedule another IEP meeting immediately.

Ms. Dow told her to wait in the office. I believed her because Ms. Dow had done that before with another aide. This action again strengthened my conviction that the woman was crazy. PaviElle had asked me earlier what was wrong with Ms. Dow. Dr. Samore saw me in the hallway and asked what was wrong. Before I could complete my story he radioed Ms. Rusch and told her I was on my way to meet with her. He also asked why Ms. Etienne was no longer with PaviElle, and was not aware of someone named Amy having been hired. When I got to Ms. Rusch's office she already had Ms. Dow in her office, so I waited outside. When I had the opportunity to speak to her I asked why after the meeting that took place the day before PaviElle had another aide. Ms. Rusch sympathized with me and promised to talk to Dr. Samore and assign Ms. Etienne to my daughter until they found a permanent aide.

My fragile emotional state of mind, which seemed to be on a wild roller coaster ride without any warning took me back to my husband's deception. I shifted my thoughts from the myriad problems at the school to Lloyd and called him crying, asking who he had called first, me or his woman, when he found out that his cousin Michael had died. He sounded surprised at my sudden question, but said emphatically, "You!" I know I must have sounded strange and confused as I proceeded to ask him if he would fall asleep when he was at his woman's house. This made him more annoyed because we both thought I was healing. He responded with, "This is bullshit. Are you going to be bringing up this matter all the time?" I did not respond, but said goodbye while I was boiling inside, trying not to explode.

This happened several times with Ms. Bradley having to make the corrections because they were all incorrect. What next, I thought. Diagnostic testing with PaviElle having several tests on the same day with no breaks. These continued issues were enough to send any weak minded human being to the asylum but I had to hold it together because my daughter was depending on me for everything.

The IEP meeting was finally held without June Eversano who had an emergency and could not attend. Dr. Samore announced that Ms. Etienne would be the permanent aide for PaviElle. He laid out a plan for all of her academic and personal needs. I was relieved but kept having lingering doubts if all this would last. I got home and stood staring through the glass doors looking at the nearby lake with tears, for the umpteenth time, flowing down my face. Also for the umpteenth time I wondered how did my life end up this way and why did PaviElle have to suffer so much and Lloyd had to cheat. I was saddened by my situation but hoping and believing that it would all be good one day in the near future.

I recalled the book I read entitled, "Living in the Now," and reminded myself to enjoy the great milestones PaviElle was showing and my husband's effort to make up for what he had done. But, I did the opposite, and instead of staying in that positive mode I spontaneously asked Lloyd for a divorce later that evening, because I no longer trusted him or felt safe with him. I could not find a good place for what he had done. I told him either PaviElle and I could go, or he could. He said he did not want a divorce and if he had to, he would kill himself. I told him he should have thought of that before he went and social studies on the recommendation of Malissa, the speech pathologist, because she thought history was too much information for her to absorb and might create an over load for her brain as it tries to recover. I asked her to double up on the time for the core subjects, math, science, language arts and regular Spanish. She agreed, and sat with me until we worked out the new schedule. As usual, we received a schedule at the end of the day that looked nothing like the one she and I had created. I dropped PaviElle off at therapy and drove back to the school to catch Ms. Rusch to let her know how upset my child was about the schedule she received. She promised to take care and solve the problem the next day and she did. This left me in a good mood especially as it was again the time of my favorite holiday, Thanksgiving.

When the New Year, 2009 arrived, the stress with school only continued. The first day of school Ms. Etienne was there as the assigned aide, but the schedule for PaviElle was just ridiculous. Some fool decided to register her in a sewing and cooking class forgetting that her left hand had Dystonia and could not function effectively. The instructor was not made aware of my daughter's condition and because she had taught her before and PaviElle had been an excellent student she gave her the sewing assignment. When PaviElle learned of the schedule she rushed to find me in Dr. Rubin's office, saying how embarrassed she felt in the class because all the work would require use of her left hand. I had to comfort her and control my emotions then find Ms. Rusch and the problem was resolved and an appropriate schedule was reinstated. Ms. Dow, on the other hand, must have had a slight reincarnation because she actually spoke closing it's doors, Janet the physical therapist that was so helpful and loved by PaviElle was off to start a new, steady job with benefits, and Malissa, the very smart speech pathologist was moving because her husband, a surgeon, had to find a new job in another state. We were devastated by these new developments.

Finding new therapists was a daunting, frustrating and extremely stressful task but I was determined to find them. After what seemed like an eternity I found a new speech therapist who was no comparison to Malissa, but we had no choice. The physical therapist replacement was so difficult Janet had to help by seeing PaviElle after work, for which I was extremely relieved and thankful. It took a very long time to find a new occupational therapist, but we eventually found Pamela. Therapy provided by the school district also continued.

It was the end of the first week of back to school and Ms. Etienne introduced us to yet another aide. Ms. Dow civility did not last long because a month later she would give PaviElle a scolding about not sitting close to the aide in class, a scolding that brought her to tears. This infuriated me so I went see Ms. Dow to ask why she was so mean to my daughter. She replied, "PaviElle is being rude to the aides and they have come crying to me also. PaviElle is not the only child in the school nor the only disabled child I have to deal with. The therapists want the aide to walk close to PaviElle but she walks fast ahead of them and when they try to help her in class she turns away her head and they consider that to be rude."

I listened to all her complaints and then asked if she knew the aide

I asked Ms. Block, the school speech pathologist to investigate if PaviElle was rude to the aide because there was no excuse for her to be rude and I would not condone that behavior. She said she would and she did.

Ms. Palmist, the new aide was a disaster. PaviElle would come home smelling of urine and when I asked why, she said the aide did not help her with getting to the toilet paper. Also when she was seeing her period she would come home with her pants and underwear soiled with blood because Ms. Palmist did not help her. I spoke to Ms. Palmist about the urine smell and bloody clothes and her attitude stunk. She took a day off and then there was yet another, Amy, followed by a Britney, then Ms. Etienne returned for a few days and yes, Ms. Palmist was the aide once more. A few weeks went by and she began to abuse PaviElle by giving her the heavy back-pack to carry along with her lunch box and heavy textbooks. Ms. Palmist also told my child "You have two hands, you can carry them." After PaviElle told me about the abuse I decided to test Ms. Palmist myself so I told PaviElle to ask her to give a message to the math teacher. She told PaviElle, "You can talk why don't you do it." I was fit to be tied and immediately went to Ms. Rusch who called in Ms. Dow. I told them about the abuse that was being endured by my daughter and demanded that they fire Ms. Palmist or remove her from being the aide. They called in Dr. Samore and he was stunned at what had happened. He pleaded with me to keep her because it was only two weeks of school left, but I said, "No way!" I told them if she was not replaced I would pull PaviElle out of school and report it to the school district. A compromise was reached and they moved rage I felt deep in my soul. In the end Ms. Etienne was the best aide PaviElle had at Okeeheelee Middle School. They bonded so well they ended the school exchanging gifts.

At graduation, PaviElle was awarded a big trophy by Dr. Samore, called the "Triumph Award," along with a very touching speech and he congratulated me for my dedication to my daughter and her recovery. She also got an award from the National Junior Honor Society and another for Spanish, with a standing ovation. This was ironic; because we had left the graduation early because PaviElle was feeling exhausted and thought she was not getting any awards. Dr. Rubin, after getting that information, called and told us to return immediately. Seeing all the students receive their awards made us both sad because PaviElle was so accustomed to being the recipient of several awards in all her previous schools, including the Principal's Award at KIPP academy. The Triumph Award was really touching because it was so unexpected and kept a secret from everyone until it was announced by Dr. Samore. The search for an appropriate high school was tedious, but my last torturous chamber came with the final IEP meeting. All the grand plans were made for high school at Palm Beach Central which has a huge campus. I listened keenly and decided to opt out of the public school system because I had done my research and found out through Susan, the school occupational therapist, that with PaviElle's disability she was qualified for the McKay Scholarship. Unfortunately, they only paid half the amount for the fees of private schools. I did everything I could possibly do to find financial help but came up blank. I then called all the private schools and discovered that they did not accept the McKay longed to hear, "Yes." I then went to Ms. Rusch and enlisted her help to complete the application process to be considered for the McKay scholarship. She graciously helped me and wished me luck. I kept monitoring the web-site to see if PaviElle was accepted.

My next challenge was to find financial aid for the other half of the tuition which we could not afford. I called my attorneys and spoke with Mr. Rosen and he advised me that there were companies that would advance me money based on the value of the ongoing medical lawsuit. I flatly refused to go that route. I persisted and wrote to several celebrities like Jill Zaren from the TV show 'New York Housewives,' because she had a daughter with JRA; Oprah, and several others, plus government agencies that told me because she was already getting the McKay scholarship she could not qualify for any other government aid. I refused to give up, so I called, Gordon, the then principal of Boca Prep but did not get him right away, but I kept calling and calling leaving several messages. On Saturday afternoon a voice said to me try calling him again and this time he answered. After apologizing for not returning the call and I explained my dilemma he said he would have to think if he could be of assistance. As I thanked him he then said, "Yes, but you will have to pay for literature books and lunch." I quickly said, "No problem. Thank you so much".

He promised to have the finance officer, Dena, give me a call to work out the exact amount and told me whatever the amount was I could pay it monthly, instead of in one payment. I was ecstatic. I called Sandra to say thanks then called Lloyd to give him the unbelievable news. God had come through again.

no problem with that decision which I would later learn was a big fat LIE. I called all the individuals at the district whose names and numbers were given to me but after leaving several voice mails and being given different names and numbers I soon concluded that I was in the midst of the phrase, "send the fool a little further."

Being the type A personality that I am, my persistence finally led me to the truth. Amy Nworb, who was now the decision point woman for me to call next. She told me the most nonsensical, ridiculous and stupid thing I have ever heard from the school district. She said, "PaviElle cannot receive the services if the private school she is attending is not a nonprofit."

I snapped and said, "Who ask if a private school is for profit or nonprofit when they enroll their child?" She was obviously speechless for a second and said, "Well, Mrs. McLaughlin that is the way the system works."

"Whomever made that decision is stupid. Thank you and goodbye,"

That afternoon my disgust for the public school churned and heightened, making me conclude that the public school system in America is totally hopeless and does not make decisions in the interest of our children whether they are disabled or able. There is help for the child that is brilliant with the "Gifted Programs," and there is free tutoring for the students who are poor, but there are no provisions or consideration for the students in the middle. This is indicative of

Deadly Negligence

of information to read and another name and number of a woman to call at the US Education Department. I called the next morning and got her voice mail. I left a message and to this day that I am writing this book I have not heard from her.

Was I disappointed, not really, because the reality is that the system is critically contaminated with incompetence, waste, misinformation and deception. You can truly only depend on yourself and God.

PaviElle began her high school journey at Boca Prep International School in August 2009 with hope and excitement. Although there had been several bumps and potholes in the road with mistakes, mishaps and reasons to be discouraged she was moving from grade to grade and improving, getting closer with God's help to be the great and successful student she once was. She fell down and hurt herself twice at school, because she no longer had a one-on-one aide or therapies that she was entitled to and needed. This occurred, ironically because of the school district's stupid decision that PaviElle would no longer receive services, designated for disabled students since she was attending a private school that was not a nonprofit organization. Keep in mind that I was told, the services would follow her to a private school, as long as I was able to get her to the therapists that were assigned.

Chapter 19

n reflection, I realized I had to train and prepare my mind in the same rigorous manner as does an athlete preparing for championships, because so arduous was the legal battle ahead. I had to celebrate all of PaviElle's milestones one by one and be encouraged that each day, God gives us at least one thing, no matter how small to show she was being restored and healed supernaturally.

The legal war raged on with James Grath, the hospital's attorney, and I went ballistic when I learned that he was trying to get the government to pay for what their hospital had inflicted upon my child. That position was quickly usurped, and the law firm wrote to say they would make all provisions to take care of her needs and recovery. For a moment I thought of the hospital making an attempt to do the right thing, but, oh, what an error of judgment I was making.

On the day of the deposition I sat face to face with Attorney James Grath at his office. The deposition I gave lasted from 10:00 a.m. to 2:30 p.m. and for my husband Lloyd, an additional 45 minutes. Grath kept harping on the drug Versed and how good a drug it can be. He

I thought if she was so gravely ill why would they give her Versed as a sleeping drug, and shouldn't the nurse have been monitoring her much more closely. Versed is a drug given to patients before an operating procedure as an anesthesia or as a sedative, and should not be given to a patient who has respiratory problems. "He is insane," I kept thinking. He kept hammering me with the same questions phrased in different ways over and over as if he was trying to break me. I remained unfazed because the truth was all I had to give.

Grath got testy when I talked about the patients in New Orleans hospitals who were given Versed to kill them during the devastating Hurricane Katrina. I tried hard to keep my composure, but couldn't help crying as I felt like the tragic incident was happening all over again. His questions took me back to the scene in the hospital. He went back and forth in an effort to confuse me and had the nerve to advise me to face reality and turn my garage that I use every day into a gym instead of what Dr. Foreman had suggested in the Life Care Plan. He said I should purchase another bicycle for PaviElle that would be more suited for her condition and face the fact that she might not improve. I told him that if I were thinking that way she would not have lived and we are not financially able just to go out and buy another bicycle. At the end of the deposition, I thought what a torture chamber I had endured with that confused man. I had to ask Mr. Rosen, my attorney, if Grath was for real as he seemed determined to make me seem like I had made a mistake or was lying about what happened to my only child. I was furious but Lloyd and Mr. Rosen tried to give me comfort. The entire weekend Lloyd and I were still reeling from the exhausting deposition. I was totally seeing and hearing Grath's voice and I could not fall asleep. I had nightmares about getting a microphone and broadcasting to all who would listen about what had happened to PaviElle. I had crazy thoughts and dreams of killing everyone from the lawyers who were digging into my medical records, trying to see if I had taken Prozac or any medication that would indicate that I was crazy, to the owners of the hospital and the big wigs in Texas who were holding the handle of the negotiations. If they were trying to come up with some fabricated legal argument that I was crazy and somehow responsible for the tragic incident that almost killed my daughter I wanted to show them that they were indeed making me crazy. Of course, God would always intervene to make me realize that I must lay all my burdens on him and he would give me rest and the justice that PaviElle deserves, because Grath's services were dismissed by the hospital after the first mediation.

When we gathered around the huge conference table in the freezing, cold room for the mediation meeting with the enemy team on one side and our team on the other, the atmosphere was filled with tension. After all the introductions were made Evon played the video that was made by a company they had hired to come to my house and videotape and interview with us and put together a short film that showed PaviElle before the brain injury and after the injury. It also showed interviews with her teachers Mr. Bender, Ms. Valdez and Dr. Rubin talking about the type of student and great achiever she was and the difficulties and challenges she now faced. All eyes were filled with tears and I was overwhelmed with so much grief that they asked if I needed to take a break. I said no because I just wanted the our daughter's recovery, especially my efforts. What was he trying to set us up for? We found out quickly as the mediator returned with a ludicrous offer made by the hospital.

I could not believe the insulting, and downright disrespectful offer they made us at mediation. Even the mediator was visibly disgusted at the offer they made and it was obvious that he told them so. He kept going back and forth and each time seemed to have gotten more and more impatient and annoyed when he could not get them to be more reasonable and willing to negotiate. I for one was in awe about the legal system in Florida that was created by President Bush when he made it law for several caps to be placed on lawsuits concerning victims suing doctors and hospitals. I kept asking what would he and his wife Laura Bush do and how much would they want if this tragic incident had happened to their beautiful twin girls who they had struggled so hard to conceive and give birth to. There was no answer because no one is concerned about a blazing fire until it is their house that is engulfed in bright orange flames.

At the end of the mediation the hospital's group of stiff and callous looking men and one slightly caring woman, seemed disheveled, drained and stressed out after, I was sure, they concluded that they were not dealing with fools or buffoons. My attorneys were just as disgusted and annoyed as Lloyd and myself, so we refused their offer and left. The ensuing months leading to another year produced more psychological torture for me. I kept praying and asking God, through his son Jesus, to take it all because I know for sure that with Him all things are possible when you believe. A new law firm was retained that turned out to be someone else's. What were they trying to do now? Lloyd who is not usually emotional like me became angry and impatient with the process and constant repeat paperwork.

They dug up our past as far as they could, trying to find out if we had sued any other entity before. That search produced a lawsuit filed by someone else who the lawyers again somehow believed was Lloyd. How desperate were they going to be to try to malign and discredit us to avoid paying for what they had done to PaviElle? Their tactics were shameful and disgraceful in my opinion. Our attorneys kept counseling us to exercise patience and go with the process. I thought the hospital's lawyers were trying to frustrate us into giving up the lawsuit and that only made me more determined to fight all the way to court, win or lose. My daughter was the important person in this equation and her suffering would not go in vain. I was not fighting for compensation for myself even though we were entitled to get it for pain and suffering, the wrecking of my family, and the state of my marriage, but I kept telling Mr. Rosen forget about me, PaviElle must be taken care of for the rest of her life. They knew I would be an excellent witness if the case went to court because I was so filled with passion, confidence and the energy to fight any battle for my

The new legal team kept asking Palm Beach County School District for PaviElle's records to prove she was a good student prior to the tragedy. Every single paperwork from all the schools she attended since kindergarten had to be submitted. I quickly figured that the new lawyers had to earn their retainer being paid to them by the

Deadly Negligence

As the legal process continued we began to feel strangled by our own financial problems and the economic crisis facing the country and our family. This led to several meltdowns by me, convincing Lloyd that we must go to counseling with Prophetess Dr. Peart, who was a religious counselor, as well as one of our pastors.

Attending church regularly gave us comfort and a place to look forward to each week so we could thank and praise God for his blessings. The counseling sessions proved to be therapeutic for us and PaviElle. We had to do several activities and read specific scriptures each night including Mark chapter 11 verses 22 to 25, and 1 John 5 verses 14 to 15. Prophetess asked me to again not bring up the subject of Lloyd's cheating, which I had eventually revealed to her, even though it was the source of much pain and heartache. I agreed, but stated that it would be difficult for me because I felt betrayed and each time Lloyd did the slightest thing to make me mad I reverted to that place of darkness. She said she understood and told us other stories that would give us encouragement.

As the weeks went by I began to feel better about Lloyd's infidelity, but was still hesitant in loosening the mortar from the bricks I had built up around my heart to prevent any further hemorrhaging. The sessions became less as Dr. Peart was convinced that we were on the road to recovery in healing and saving our marriage and family. I was relieved that PaviElle finally had a voice and a chance to express her feelings and hurt in counseling by simply saying "I am mad and angry with Dad because he hurt mommy." I could visibly see her relief and a weight off her young shoulders. She was only 15 years old and

The anticipation of the outcome of the lawsuit was killing me. The next event in this saga was to attend a pre-mediation meeting at Mr. Rosen's office. He also wanted to introduce new attorney, Bill Wolk, who had been added to our team, as well as another attorney, a woman who specialized in trusts, something we were required by law to set up for our daughter's well being. Bill was a great addition; I liked him immediately and he turned out to be a very smart, valuable voice for our legal team. The female attorney, Mephanie Snyderman, rattled my spirit from the start and I was totally unhappy that she had the nerve to charge us for coming to sell us her services. I was convinced to use her because she was good at her chosen specialty of law and was the only available and the least expensive attorney in town. I accepted her services, but this would prove in the end not to be that great as she proved to be disorganized and extremely confrontational and disrespectful.

There were moments I wanted to dismiss her because I felt she was displaying signs of distrust, disrespect and even racism towards us. Mr. Rosen had to be the voice of reason, the great lawyer and human being he is, and advised me that it would be a mistake to retain a new lawyer. I reluctantly agreed and we pressed forward.

The mediation with the hospital's new law firm appeared at first to be more compassionate and respectful until they came up with yet another insulting offer. "Are these people insane or what?" I kept asking myself. Our financial advisor for our team suggested they send me to speak to the hospital attorneys with the passion I obviously had for what had happened to my daughter. He also said that he

The battle continued and the hurdles became higher only causing us more frustration and anxiety in our lives. PaviElle's financial need for extra tutoring was increasing and we needed extra money to provide for her so she would not fall behind.

Another year would pass before mediation was scheduled and this time I was ready for whatever the hospital's legal team was bringing in their bag of legal and numbers trickery. I was given several scriptures to read by Pastor Fred in the book of Psalms. I had put on the whole armor of God and felt this was the day for justice to prevail. I in turn gave all the scriptures to Lloyd and told him to read them every day. We decided to stand strong and firm against the devil because I believed with all my heart and soul that Satan is a big lie and he can only play his hand if you allow him into your life and circle.

Even while I was sitting at the table during the mediation I was reading the Psalms on my cell phone. I read so much that my battery died and when it was time to call PaviElle to tell her we were still at the mediation table and I had made arrangements for Clement, my friend Judy's husband, to pick her up as he had to pass her school to go home, I had to borrow Evon's cell phone to make the call. Lloyd's phone was also dead.

After strong and sometimes tense negotiations our legal battle came to an end but it would take several months for PaviElle to get the financial help she so desperately needed. God came through, but I was very emotional and told my team of lawyers that, "The hospital and their powerful legal team had gotten away with murder."

I was told by the only female on our legal team about a teenage boy's case that she worked on, prior to joining Rosen and Rosen, who could barely do anything for himself and the settlement he got at trial was abysmal. I felt sick to my stomach for days and suffered with remorse, doubt and haunting questions about the decision I had agreed to for my girl. I had to pray and ask God each day to help me accept and feel better about my decision.

I called Bill Wolk, one of my attorney's, and he revealed to me that he was struggling with the same thoughts until he called some of his peers and they told him the decision was best for everyone and would save us from a long arduous trial with no guarantees at the end, and which would have taken several years and place unnecessary stress on our family. At the end of that phone call I did not bother to call Mr. Rosen or Evon who were next on my mind to discuss how I was struggling emotionally with the decision that was made.

Bill made me feel much better and followed through on all the different things we had to do, including another attorney appointed by the court to make sure we were comfortable with the settlement and the procedure going forward. This came with its own set of issues and going to court for a second time to stand before the judge who did not make eye contact or recognize our presence was a little disturbing for me. I started to cry so hard when he tried to question certain things that Mr. Rosen had to get tissue and try to console me. This was just awkward and devastating and totally crushed my feelings. Then there was the female trust attorney again at the final day in court where she treated us like we were her underlings who was required and get the case rapped up immediately. I no longer communicated with her or her office and it became clear that she was acting like a Gestapo agent who was put in charge of us. I kept asking if she had forgotten that we were paying her and she was working for us not the other way around.

I could continue writing more and more pages about an unimaginable experience that my only child had to endure, suffer through and could only recover from with the supernatural powers of God in the name of his son Jesus. Getting through all the fights with Medicaid, and finding therapists that were the best at their profession, was an extremely stressful and sometimes disappointing journey, but God gave me strength when I thought I had none left, courage to fight for all the things that PaviElle was entitled to, and search through the complicated maze to find things that were available free of cost and good. Through all the pain and sorrow it was always a celebration for every milestone that PaviElle achieved each day.

Some days brought laughter and others produced tears of joy like the day she received an invitation from NJHS to the honor roll festivities of which she was a member every year. I congratulated her and touched her face because I could not hug her while trying to keep driving in the traffic. I remembered the morning she ran into my room, very excited because she managed to put her bra on for the first time in years. She dressed herself and was so proud in spite of the struggle. I also remembered the evening she felt overwhelmed with the amount of school work she had to complete and as I tried to assist her with arranging her notebook she got upset and said, "You

Park on a school trip when she got sick and I had to pick her up and bring her ginger ale, then she returned to Jenine, her golf coach, for lessons and did very well.

I remembered the Sunday morning she came to my room and gave me a big hug and I told her the cream I used on her face was finished and that we needed to find a dermatologist to get some more. She said to me, "Call me, I could mix something up today." I laughed and gave her another hug. It was clear her memory of wanting to become a dermatologist since she was younger had been restored.

Then there was the report from Janet that she was proud to see PaviElle go up the hill backwards and climbed the ladder by herself, and Malissa's report that she was doing fractions so well and asking me what I was doing with her to have this success so quickly. I told her we were at it every single day. And, the morning she woke up early and began sketching just like she did in the past. Our thanks and shout for joy when she screamed, "Look mom!" When we looked we saw her left hand was flat on the bed instead of being hooked at the wrist. We hugged real tight and kept shouting, praising and giving God the glory. She was also regaining the admiration of boys at school and how proud she felt because students were asking her for help with math the way it was as far back as KIPP Academy in Atlanta. She was sneaking to call her friends on the cell phone early in the mornings, but when I found out and told her that was not accepted she refused to take her cell phone back to school. She was beginning to be a teenager again. Trying to make her own cereal and putting it in the microwave and setting the cooking time; being able to drink from a straw and writing me notes of apology when she laces. This was especially gratifying because she had now relearned the skills necessary to completely dress herself although it was at a very slow pace and required patience. Buttoning her shirt was exhilarating and so was brushing her hair and putting in scrunches to tie her ponytail. The ability to take a shower without my help have no words to describe, along with shaving her under arms and legs. Scoring a 91 on a history test in the first quarter of 11th grade filled her heart and soul with pride, joy, self confidence, self-esteem and a renewed faith in God's supernatural powers. This also encouraged her to take my advice and read Jabez prayer, 1 Chronicles chapter 4:10, every day and see what God does. " And Jabez called on the God of Israel, saying, Oh that thou wouldest bless me indeed, and enlarge my coast, and that thine hand might be with me, and that thou wouldest keep me from evil, that it may not grieve me! And God granted him that which he requested."

Washing her first plate and mastering sharing her own meal excited her and she longed for the day she could cook and help me bake again. Learning to drive the golf cart with Lloyd and then finally able to be the sole driver with dad riding behind her has played a great role in restoring her self confidence and self esteem. The smile on her face as she told me about her accomplishment was priceless and skyrocketed hope.

She has come to terms with the tragedy that occurred in her life, and is accepting words from the Bible that God has a way of turning what was meant for evil into good. I believed that PaviElle's greatest joy and self confidence booster was her hair that had grown back her ability to dance with rhythm and being invited to Prophetess's house for Thanksgiving in 2008 and 2009 where she felt her social abilities were restored.

It is with great regret that this tradition had to come to an end because of one insecure individual's jealousy, disrespect and downright rudeness shown to my family that made us decide never to return to celebrate this holiday and save us the hurt feelings and disappointment. This decision really gave us great pause but it had to be made to restore our self-respect and dignity of not being insulted at someone's home, not by the gracious and beautiful homeowner but by someone else who she obviously adores and can never get rid of. We felt somewhat better when we realized this person had offended several others and is consumed with insecurity and jealousy. It was also special for PaviElle to attend Judy's birthday party and being honored with a special prayer and celebrated for being so determined to get better and return to being a normal teenager. Her occupational therapist, Teri, told her constantly that she admired her courage to never QUIT at any task she gave in therapy sessions. PaviElle's ultimate joy was going on her first cruise to Nassau, Bahamas on Norwegian Cruise line over the summer of 2011. She enjoyed the cruise so much that when we returned to Miami she said. "I wish we were turning back to go again." Her 18th birthday celebration will be another cruise, a wish that will fill her heart and be well deserved for all the suffering and pain she has endured for the past four years. She is also now able to face any bully at school, like a boy name Kevin, and stand up and speak up for herself. There are several hurdles left in my daughter's journey trusting and believing in God with unwavering faith and hope. She is now wanting to be a perfumier, dessert bakery entrepreneur and learning to drive a car and not just the golf cart.

Chapter 20

his tragic journey with my daughter's illness and my marital challenges has taught me numerous lessons. For one, and painfully, I have learned that friends are never who you think they are, because in times of your most desperate life experiences only the genuinely true friends stay for the long journey. It is, however, possible for you to find new friends in the midst of your walk through the valley of the Shadow of death, but they also eventually fall by the wayside. I know for sure that God places people in your life for different reasons and purposes and you must be prepared when that ends without trying to hold on.

I was fortunate to find such a friend in friendship with the Prophetess. Meeting her came through a divine connection and no matter what happens or whichever demonic spirit tries to break up our friendship, or come between us in some way, our friendship and love for each other remain strong. Sometimes the nurturing of the friendship is difficult, mostly on her side because of time constraints, but I will always believe that not having time shouldn't be used as the reason for not connecting with a friend and nurturing that friendship. We have certainly have had great highs and low points in our friendship from anyone, or friend, who caused me any level of hurt, but there is just no answer to that question but divine connection. Unfortunately this truth may have come to an end because there have been so many excuses on her part just to make time. I have come to the conclusion and told her that she is too important and busy to nurture a friendship that is truly filled with true love, loyalty, care and a willingness to make time for the other person. She disagrees but nothing has changed and I am sure that God is the only source if there is going to be reconciliation, apologies and dedication, or will it be a part of the journey that comes to an end through all the pain and twists, turns and disappointments of my life. It will be difficult to come to grips with this but truly only God knows what the future holds and miracles do happen. I will continue to wait for this miracle because of my deep love for her.

My husband who I loved and trusted completely disappointed me in an inexplicable way. I am not sure that my pain, and my heart, that was broken into so many little pieces, can be totally repaired, but I have made a conscious decision to continue to pray hard and doing the best I possibly can to dig deep down into my soul and find that love again, along with the trust. I struggle each day to keep my mind and thoughts away from his sordid affair, but I still believe the stubborn memories that remain stems from my conviction that the affair began and continued even when PaviElle laid dying in a hospital and I was at the most vulnerable point, emotionally, in my life.

While in the process of writing this book a clear voice came to me trust we had can never be rebuilt but he always insisted that our marriage will work and there will be no divorce or separation. I have come to a good place in my heart especially on the days when Lloyd is being nice or showing he cares, so I will continue to dream big and pray very hard. Dealing with the timing of the affair was clearly the most difficult, and keeps me sometimes asking why, and always concerned about the long term effect it will have on PaviElle when she finds love and marry.

She made me laugh so hard recently when I was talking to Lloyd on the car telephone about being more romantic and showing affection. She listened and said "I will help you daddy" but after a moment she said "No I will not help you I am saving my ideas for my own person."

We laughed so hard I almost missed my exit to home from the highway. My heart was so filled with joy and I realized she has got her humorous personality back with the ability to think on her feet. I have also learned a profound lesson that when you make a decision to get married and have children they become the center of your life and if and when misfortune comes you must be prepared to give up all your dreams because their life comes before yours at all times.

I have also come to know God in a way that can never be shaken. I trust, believe, hope, have complete faith without doubt, and know for sure that with God, and through his son Jesus, all things are possible. It is also clear to me that church, no matter how great it seems, and your belief that God wants you to assemble with other brethren, can be filled with workers of iniquity who are merely one day Christians prophetesses, and other church leaders. If you are new to a church congregation beware, because no matter what expertise, financial input, or promotion you are able to provide for the church, the old members who are accustomed to sit on their butts and do nothing, will cut you down like a wood chopper cutting down an oak tree. I had to make sure that I was always covered with the blood of Jesus, and total armor of God, keeping my guard up and developing a spine of steel in order to absorb the insults, sometimes subtle and other times blatant as I tried to make a genuine contribution to the church I joined.

My expectation that people in church are somehow converted to Christ, and accordingly would behave better than the non-converted population was dashed by the high level of hypocrisy that I found rampant among some members of the congregation. The constant hustle to see who can get and maintain all the love, care and attention from the church leaders was shocking and extremely surprising, In the midst of witnessing seemingly great miracles in the church, the lack of discipline, selfishness and great secrecy and conniving among members and leaders was appalling. When I questioned the uncertain feelings I was experiencing I was told that church is like a hospital and those who come there are people who are seeking healing but some take a much longer time to receive that healing while others grab it quickly, and then there are those that will need God to come and grab them by the throat for them to be healed, converted and change their wicked ways.

It was also interesting to observe the young people, especially, showcase their talents and sell their multilevel marketing schemes to unwitting innocent suckers who are chasing the get-rich-quick

I was also struck by the level of nepotism and display of bias tendencies, that was rampant in the church, leaving some members to be constantly stewing, but not willing or able to face their fears and express their concerns about the problem, for fear of losing the love or special place they think they have in a leader's heart. They fight for positions and leadership roles that most of them are neither qualified nor capable of completing; they continue to crave special tasks even when they constantly display nothing but incompetence. Also, I was shocked to observe there were members in the church who are indeed capable, usually showing competence and reliability but because of their weakness and fear of speaking up for what's right and their obvious insecurities in trying not to lose their closeness to the leader, are denied the opportunity to serve.

Then there are those in the church who seem entrenched in their belief that everything that happens in their lives is the result of someone working witchcraft, or always blamed on the devil. They seem to have the inability to look in the mirror, see themselves and ask what did they do to bring the devil into their lives, or if their belief in the workers of Iniquity was controlling their subconscious

I will never again allow myself to be a member of a church where I face disrespect, am accosted and attacked on several occasions to

Deadly Negligence

and animosity towards you is justified in the minds of some insecure members, as they try to convince themselves that you are sharing your ideas and your efforts to take over their church, without consideration that you have no such interest.

Maybe the church I am looking for does not exist. but I will keep looking and hoping that God will reveal to me that special place or take that special leader and give him or her the knowledge to create an environment that will weed out some of the thorns, and be strong and inspirational enough to change the hearts of the problem members and transform them to be more Christ-like, accommodating, willing to share The love and prophetic words they may have within them. This, I am convinced, will allow churches to be more receptive to, and grow with new members who join those churches and are willing to roll up their sleeves, work hard without seeking accolades, but strive to serve God in a very pure and humble manner without the distraction of the envy and what some refer to as "curry favor." As the famous author, Louise Hale, said "I'd rather be loved for who I am than loved for whom I am not."

I believe, and am assured, that all I want for PaviElle, Lloyd, my mom and myself is already here, because I have created in my mind through the power of visualization all that my heart desires. It is God's promise, something I keep in mind, that He will give us the POWER not only to create wealth, but also to believe and trust Him to give us the desires of our hearts. We must also understand that through all our suffering and pain there is always a rainbow that shows up after the rain pours and the sunshine begins to shine no more." When the doctor gave me the diagnosis from my blood work I simply got angry. I began to explain to him my lifestyle and what I had gone through in my life with my daughter and husband, but he held my hands and said, "You will be fine."

I next did my annual mammogram at the usual imaging company thinking all would be well as my tests always were, but later got a telephone call on my way to pick up my daughter from school. The uncaring voice on the phone said I had to schedule another appointment to do more pictures and an ultra sound. As my heart began to race I asked why, but the woman on the phone said I had to call my doctor.

After she confirmed the appointment and hung up I immediately called my doctor's office and asked to speak to the nurse. I asked her why I had to do more tests and she explained that the mammogram was incomplete so I needed to do more photos, but there was nothing to worry about. When I hung up the phone I asked myself how she could say there was nothing to worry about when the woman who called sounded so panicked with a tone of urgency. I began to pray and rebuke whatever they saw, asking God to spear me from anymore suffering. I prayed hard and invoked all the scriptures of healing I had relied on with my child, but I told no one what was happening. I kept praying and praying, then the next morning I got a call from Pastor Fred, who asked, "Sister Diana are you OK?" I told him I was, but he kept asking me if I was sure as I didn't sound like I had the enthusiasm I usually had. With him sensing I had a problem, I told him of my fears and he explained that the Spirit had told him

Deadly Negligence   251

was long and stressful but I kept my thoughts positive, looking around the room wondering what all the other patients were there to find out.

The clerk who called my name was extremely pleasant and caring so I complemented her and told her she had chosen the right profession. She thanked me and proceeded with all the paperwork and the billing process. Coincidentally, there was another lady in the waiting room whose name was also Diana. When the radiologist came out and called, "Diana" we both got up and everyone in the waiting room looked at us. We both asked the clerk if there was a mistake and she said, there was no mistake, as there were definitely two Diana's present. I was directed to the locker room, given a gown to put on and sent to another waiting room. There I again met, and introduced myself to the other Diana, a tall gorgeous, elegant woman who told me she had breast cancer. She told me how she felt when the doctor gave her the diagnosis seven years ago and that she was currently a breast cancer survivor. She explained that everyone asked her about her treatment and survival, but it was not easy to explain because the treatment for the disease has changed and improved so much in the past seven years. She explained how her husband wanted to support her so he decided to be with her at her follow up mammograms even though she kept telling him he did not have to. Her husband persisted and she agreed but he almost fainted as he observed the pressure and tight squeeze on the
breast as the test was done. She advised me to listen to my doctor and express my feelings, but to always take someone with me when I went to hear the diagnosis. As I was called to do my test I held her

finished she told me she had to take the picture to the doctor to see if he needed more images so I had to wait in the room again. Then came the ultra sound technician who was soft spoken and gentle. As she began that exam I kept asking her what she was seeing and she said she only saw an extremely small nodule. Hearing her tone of voice I knew for sure God had answered my prayer because I could endure nothing more. I explained to her that I did regular breast exams and she assured me that self-examination would never reveal a nodule so small. My anxiety subsided and I stopped questioning myself about not finding this by myself.

When I returned to my doctor I asked if the cold manner in which I was informed that I had to do another mammogram was the norm. I told him that healthcare professionals should be more considerate about their patients' emotions especially when they were being given adverse news about diagnostic tests like mammograms that were related to the possibility of having a disease like cancer. He apologized on behalf of the staff of the imaging center, but reminded me that although I was called to redo the test he had initially told me I had nothing to worry about. The outcome of this experience has increased my faith in God and his son Jesus, and my conviction that prayers are answered.

I have also learned that I am intolerant and tired of hearing the words, "I'm Sorry." It would be so much better not hearing excuses and be saved from any more hypocrisy. I have grown tired of hearing people saying what they think you want to hear instead of saying what they mean. Making excuses for not spending time with the ones one day Christians who believe they are superior and more in tune with God. I'll now reveal the scriptures I read in the hospital daily for healing, restoration and expectation:

> Psalms 118 vs. 6,
> Psalms 107 vs. 20,
> Psalms 103 vs. 2 and 3,
> Psalms 30 vs. 2,
> Psalms 46 vs. 1 to 3,
> 1 Peter, Chapter 2 vs. 24
> Third John 2,
> Galatians 3 – 4,
> Isaiah 53 vs. 5,
> Jeremiah 30 vs. 17,
> Exodus 15 – 26, 23 – 25,
> Matthew 9 – 35

For believing and hope, Psalms 30 vs. 5, and Psalms 37 vs. 3 to 8.

For healing my marriage and family, Mark 11, 23 and 24, 1 John 5, 14 and 15.

For the legal struggles and mediations: All the verses of Psalms 3, 4, 5, 17, 18, 20, 21, 23, 25, 36, 46, 55, 62, 69, 102, 103, 107, 109.

Writing this book has been very therapeutic for me, although there were several days I thought I just could not continue to dredge up the pain, suffering and devastation I felt when these unfortunate experiences began. But, on the emotional days that I kept crying, I personal feelings as a contribution to this book, so they can also Benefit from the therapeutic cleansing I have experienced.

No matter how things are going and no matter what many people think of her, PaviElle always says this, "I'll do me, and you do you." The following is her message:

"Every day I enjoy life and what God has blessed me with. I still ask God, 'When is your miracle going to be complete?' I know HE doesn't rush things but since I am a teenager, I feel at times out of place with the other kids at school since I had to do my 8th grade year over again, because I got sick for that whole year in which I was supposed to go into 8th grade. I contemplate and wish I have a "Do Over" in life, but I can't, God does things for a reason I guess. I should have been a senior this year but instead I am a junior. When I look at all my friends going into 12th grade I feel so bad, but I try to remain focused and in faith." (PaviElle).

Reading what PaviElle has written made me cry, feeling a deep sense of sadness so I used this as an opportunity to explain again, why I made the decision to have her repeat 8th grade although she had passed it with flying colors.

I explained that the school wanted her to go to 9th grade but because of the brain injury she had suffered it would be better for her to go back to a grade she had already mastered in an environment where she already knew all the teachers and the school itself, instead of being in a new school with all new teachers and new material to knowing that everywhere we go everyone thinks she is twelve years old.

The following are the thoughts my mom, Crysel, placed into words:

"One of the darkest days of my life was when I received a call stating that a disobedient nurse had administered a life threatening medication to my granddaughter PaviElle. Suddenly I experienced an innermost pain and emptiness. I became numb with inexplicable emotions. I recalled all the precious moments my granddaughter and I spent together, the little things she said, the sincere love she showed me, our bonding moments and so much more. As I observed her pain and suffering, I felt so helpless and confused. In my confusion it dawned on me that 'GOD IS ABLE.' I began praying to God asking for his deliverance, healing and blessings. I gave it all to JESUS. I thought that I should bring my wounded heart, my troubled soul and tell my anguish to God in prayer. I thought one has no sorrow that heaven cannot heal."

As I confided in our Father I began experiencing peace and healing for my wounded heart. Over time some of my actions have changed. I moan and complain less. I am appreciating each moment much more, thanking God for every blessing. I take nothing for granted; I try to be more patient, less angry and more understanding of other people's pain. My daughter and I have a better relationship. We communicate more sensibly and show more understanding for each other's feelings. We laugh more and are more accepting of each other's shortcomings.

God holds the future. I am giving loving thanks for the Lord's lavish gifts, they are many and they are great. My thought process has changed and I give thanks continuously." (Crysel).

Lloyd took the longest time to state his feelings about PaviElle's tragedy but this is what he wrote:

"Thursday morning June 7, 2007 preparing for the day's work schedule like I always do, making sure I had the required materials to complete schedule customers appointments, my telephone rang.

Before I could say hello my wife screamed, 'They killed our daughter, they killed our daughter.' I replied 'What?' 'They killed our daughter,' she repeated. Then I heard a voice in the background that said, 'No she is not dead.' I knew something was seriously wrong so my priorities were immediately redirected.

Upon arrival at the hospital I dashed to the PICU, my wife's face was washed in tears and she appeared to be too weak to speak. I proceeded to PaviElle's room. When I got to her room door, 'Oh my God!' I exclaimed, my knees buckled, eyes filled with tears, my whole body became weak and I was unable to stand. I was not prepared for what I saw. I felt saddened and angry yet this ordeal had taught me humility. We do not know what is going to take place the next second, minute or hour, so we should not miss out on the moments that gives life meaning." (Lloyd).

I hope that after reading this book everyone will know that it does

I could have chosen to stay angry at the hospital, doctors and that nurse for ruining my only child's life, the extremely long road of recovery, and my husband for cheating on me at the lowest point in my life. Instead I made the choice to forgive, grow in my faith and know that you can always conquer and overcome anything that happens to you in your journey of life.

May you truly believe as God truly blesses you. *Diana*

Epilogue

fter five years of a journey that has changed my outlook on life in a way that no one could have dreamed, anticipated, predicted, wanted or needed, my hope in God's miracles is stronger than ever. I now rely on all of God's promises and focus each day on the scripture of Joel chapter 2, verse 25 that says, "And I will restore to you the years that the locust hath eaten, the cankerworm, and the caterpillar, and the palmer worm, my great army which I sent among you". Verse 26: "And ye shall eat in plenty and be satisfied, and praise the name of the Lord your God, that hath dealt wondrously with you and my people shall never be ashamed."

I also focus on God's words in Daniel chapter 3, verse 16: "Shadrach, Meshach and Abednego, answered and said to the king, O Nebuchadnezzar, we are not careful to answer thee in this matter." Verse 17: "If it be so, our God whom we serve is able to deliver us from the burning fiery furnace, and he will deliver us out of thine hand, O king."

My intention is to help everyone to Love themselves the way they are wonderfully made by God. Parents must teach their children to Love a burning fiery furnace without hurt, then I know for sure that he will deliver me from the catastrophic events in my life; he will totally restore PaviElle and, hopefully, my marriage.

Recently, I had such a meltdown I woke Lloyd at 4:00 a.m. to let him know that I am angry and I want my life back. This includes wanting my daughter's life back, my career and my marriage, so the healing process is ongoing. When I watch her struggle to open the refrigerator, put her hair in a ponytail, put on her pantyhose and just take care of her daily functions it still breaks my heart. I also know that when I freaked out that morning it was the first time Lloyd really understood the hurt and pain that I was feeling or have been feeling for these four years. I have also learned to bury Lloyd's affair, but like burying your loved one or friend on the day of a funeral their goodness or faults you still remember. During the 2011 holiday season Lloyd finally told me he was very angry with himself for what he had done.

I am very happy and thankful that PaviElle is doing well in school with all her disabilities and what she lost with the brain injury. My marriage is on the mend and I hope and expect that my career can restart with the promotion of this book and possible speaking engagements as PaviElle regains her independence and relies on me less. This is a long look down the future road but I know God with his supernatural powers can change all things immediately, and with him all things are possible.

Friendships have become more difficult even with those I thought there was a divine connection with, because people always have what the Bible says:"In all things guard your heart."

Over the years my attitude has protected me from heartbreaks with men, and a loss of self with friends. I have never wanted to be anyone else but who God made me to be and that is the reason I wrote and produced a rap music song titled "I Love Me". Deep in my heart and soul I know our lives will be good, filled with joy and happiness in the future and telling this story about this devastating near death experience of my daughter, PaviElle, will help families somewhere in the world giving them strength to continue, and enable them to put their natural with God's supernatural and believe that miracles do happen.

In the beginning of this tragic journey I wrote my declaration and placed it over her hospital bed. It stated "PaviElle is Totally Healed in the name of Jesus" Now I Declare and Decree that " PaviElle will be TOTALLY Restored with a Genius Brain and Genius memory with exceptional success, prosperity, peace, happiness and joy in her life in the name of Jesus." AMEN.

BOOKS ARE AVAILABLE AT:
WWW.AMAZON.COM
DIANAWRIGHTTV.WEBS.COM
WWW.SIXHEARTSPUBLISHING.COM

PLEASE ORDER YOUR COPY TODAY AND TAKE A STAND AGAINST 'DEADLY NEGLIGENCE AND HOSPITAL ERRORS'

Printed in Great Britain
by Amazon.co.uk, Ltd.,
Marston Gate.